Practical Approach to Peripheral Arterial Chronic Total Occlusions

Subhash Banerjee

Editor

Practical Approach to Peripheral Arterial Chronic Total Occlusions

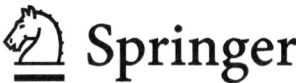 Springer

Editor
Subhash Banerjee
University of Texas Southwestern Medical Center
Dallas, Texas, USA

ISBN 978-981-10-3052-9   ISBN 978-981-10-3053-6   (eBook)
DOI 10.1007/978-981-10-3053-6

Library of Congress Control Number: 2017936690

Printed on acid-free paper

This Springer imprint is published by Springer Nature
The registered company is Springer Nature Singapore Pte Ltd.
The registered company address is: 152 Beach Road, #21-01/04 Gateway East, Singapore 189721, Singapore

Preface

This book is written to provide cardiovascular specialists with the tools to complete endovascular interventions of lower extremity peripheral artery occlusions with purpose and confidence. Effective information management and swift clinical decision-making play a powerful role in the life of an endovascular specialist. Acquiring chronic total occlusion (CTO) intervention skills in a systematic and reproducible manner need not be such a grueling and arduous task. With the right approach and comprehensive knowledge of specific tools, tackling peripheral artery CTOs can be rewarding for both the operator and the patient. During my years as a clinical and academic physician, training the next generation of endovascular specialists, I have watched operators initially daunted by the complexity and diversity CTO lesions grow to master this technically challenging procedure. With its step-by-step methodical approach, this book and its contents are designed to familiarize the reader with the current aspects of peripheral artery CTO intervention techniques and enable them to effortlessly bridge the gap in mastering this challenging, yet common, medical procedure.

Dallas, TX, USA   Subhash Banerjee

Acknowledgment and Dedication

First and foremost, I would like to thank my wife, Pooja, for her relentless support and encouragement throughout the course of my entire career. Her strength has allowed me to seek the knowledge and opportunities without which I would not be the man, father, or physician I am today. For that, I dedicate this book to her.

Next, my children Avantika (Sonu) and Rahul, for never failing to make me smile and being understanding of the many nights and mornings I have had to spend away from home or working on this book. My parents, for allowing me to pursue my dreams and ambitions from childhood, and my family, especially Kiki and Shivani, for believing in and supporting me at the most primitive stages of my career.

My friend and colleague Dr. Emmanouil Brilakis (Manos), my mentor Dr. Joseph Hill, and my coauthors for having supplied me with the knowledge, wisdom, and opportunities that were able to make this book come to fruition. Thank you to the community of cardiovascular specialists and to my patients who have continually been the source of timeless inspiration throughout the course of my life.

Contents

Chapter 1
Medical Management of Lower Extremity Peripheral Artery Disease

Akshar Y. Patel and Hitinder S. Gurm

1.1 Introduction

An estimated 8–12 million Americans are believed to suffer from peripheral arterial disease (PAD) according to the American Heart Association [1]. The prevalence of PAD has been estimated at almost 10% in the general population and almost 20% in those older than 70 years. Patients with PAD present a unique challenge to the provider due to their typically older age, high rates of underdiagnosis due to asymptomatic state, and the higher prevalence of comorbid conditions. The prototypical risk factors for PAD are similar to that of coronary arterial disease and include tobacco use, hyperlipidemia, hypertension, and diabetes. The mainstay of PAD therapy is aggressive risk factor modification followed by pharmacologic therapy and exercise therapy as warranted.

1.2 Risk Factor Modification

1.2.1 Tobacco Use

Though cigarette smoking is quite well known as risk factor for other cardiovascular conditions, it has the absolute strongest correlation with PAD. Tobacco use is the largest risk factor for PAD with epidemiological studies demonstrating up to a sixfold increased risk of the development of PAD in patients who

A.Y. Patel, MD • H.S. Gurm, MD (✉)
Department of Medicine, Samuel and Jean A. Frankel Cardiovascular Center,
University of Michigan Health System and Medical School, Ann Arbor, MI, USA

VA Ann Arbor Health Care, Ann Arbor, MI, USA
e-mail: hgurm@med.umich.edu

© Springer Science+Business Media Singapore 2017
S. Banerjee (ed.), *Practical Approach to Peripheral Arterial Chronic Total Occlusions*, DOI 10.1007/978-981-10-3053-6_1

smoke tobacco; furthermore, this risk has been demonstrated to be dose dependent on the amount of tobacco use [2]. Moreover, once a patient has been diagnosed with PAD, the continued use of cigarettes has been directly related to the progression of PAD and eventual limb loss. This effect is also seen in an attenuation of response with the use of pharmacologic and endovascular interventions in the PAD patient who continues to use cigarettes [3]. Studies have also demonstrated an increased dose-dependent risk of PAD development in patients who do not smoke cigarettes themselves but are a victim of secondhand smoke exposure [4]. More recently, e-smoking has been increasing in popularity due to perceived lower-risk profile; though conclusive studies on e-smoking's risk on PAD do not exist, there are some concerns that the perceived benefits of e-smoking may be outweighed by greater vapor and secondhand exposure in regard to PAD risk [5].

1.2.2 Hyperlipidemia, Hypertension, and Diabetes

Well-known lipid risk factors for PAD include elevated low-density lipoprotein (LDL), elevated triglycerides, low high-density lipoprotein, and lipoprotein (a) [6]. Hypertension has been demonstrated to be a risk factor for PAD development in many long-standing population studies. In Framingham, men were two times as likely and women four times as likely to develop PAD with intermittent claudication if they were hypertensive [7]. Similarly, in the Cardiovascular Health Study patients with a history hypertension were noted to have a 50% greater likelihood of the development of PAD [8]. While tobacco use typically results in PAD in the larger inflow vessels of the extremities, diabetes mellitus as a risk factor typically results in PAD in the more distal vessels. A large meta-analysis has demonstrated that with every one-percent increase in A1c greater than six, there is a 30% increased risk for the incidence of PAD [9]. Moreover, diabetics who develop PAD are known to suffer five times higher risk of amputation compared to nondiabetics with PAD [10]. As such, the control of risk factors in even those patients who have already developed PAD is an important part of the therapeutic plan.

1.3 Therapeutics: Control of Risk Factors and CV Mortality and Morbidity

The primary goals of therapy for PAD include the prevention of myocardial infarction, stroke, and death as well as prevention of limb loss and avoidance of surgery or endovascular procedures.

1.3.1 Smoking Cessation Therapy

Smoking cessation is a key therapy for patients with PAD. Numerous studies have demonstrated objective improvements in ankle pressures and walking distance as well as reductions in need for limb amputations with tobacco cessation [11, 12]. The treatment options for smoking cessation are varied but almost always include a component of behavior-modification therapies including counseling and/or support groups. Such behavior-modification therapies alone have been demonstrated as having 20% efficacy at 1 year in eliminating tobacco use [13]. Nicotine supplementation is also often used with an efficacy of close to 50% seen at 1 year [14]. Short-term pharmacologic options include varenicline and bupropion, both of which have been approved by the FDA for assistance in smoking cessation; they have demonstrated 40% and 35% efficacies, respectively, at 1 year [15, 16]. The American Heart Association and the American College of Cardiology provide a Class I (A) recommendation to both advise for smoking cessation at each clinic visit as well as offer comprehensive cessation options for all patients with PAD [17].

1.3.2 Lipid Lower Therapy with Statins

Though specific levels for PAD have not been separately stated in the guidelines, as a CAD equivalent, similar goals of LDL <70 mg/dL for high-risk patients have been used; the utilization of statins provides a benefit with respect to reduction in myocardial infarction, stroke, and vascular death rates. A Cochrane meta-analysis found no change in ABI but did show increase in total walking distance (152 m) and pain-free walking distance (90 m) with statin use in patients with PAD [18].

1.3.3 Hypertension Control with Angiotensin-Converting Enzyme Inhibition

Though the control of hypertension by any antihypertensive is beneficial in reducing the risk of PAD and vascular disease in general, angiotensin-converting enzyme inhibitors have been shown to have a mortality benefit. The HOPE trial demonstrated a reduction in myocardial infarction, stroke, and vascular death for patients with PAD treated with an angiotensin-converting enzyme inhibitors; this benefit was seen even if there was no reduction in blood pressure [19]. Furthermore, a study comparing ramipril versus placebo demonstrated functional improvement with an improved pain-free walking time (75 s longer) and maximum walking time (255 s longer) [20].

1.3.4 Antiplatelet Therapy

Aspirin, the prototypical antiplatelet drug for vascular disease, has been shown to provide a 23% reduction in major vascular events including myocardial infarction, stroke, and vascular death in patients with PAD [21]. Similarly, patients with PAD on low-dose aspirin therapy have demonstrated a 54% reduction in the risk of the morbidity of peripheral vascular surgery [22]. The CAPRIE trial advanced antiplatelet therapy further by evaluating the P2Y12 inhibitor, clopidogrel, against aspirin therapy in PAD patients; it demonstrated a 24% reduction in the risk of myocardial infarction, stroke, and vascular death [23]. The CHARISMA trial attempted to demonstrate a benefit in dual-antiplatelet therapy (aspirin and clopidogrel) over aspirin-only therapy. However, though secondary analyses did demonstrate a major cardiovascular outcomes benefit for dual-antiplatelet therapy in a composite of patients with prior myocardial infarction, prior stroke, and prior PAD, it failed to demonstrate a statistically significant difference in those patients with only prior PAD [24]. As such, the current American College of Cardiology and American Heart Association guidelines provide for a Class I recommendation of clopidogrel alone with a Class IIb recommendation for clopidogrel and aspirin dual-antiplatelet therapy as a reasonable more intensive therapeutic option in those patients who warrant it [17].

1.4 Therapeutics: Improvement of Functional Capacity

The secondary goal of PAD therapy is to improve functional capacity and symptoms including pain-free activities, walking ability, and the delaying of limb amputation (Fig. 1.1).

1.4.1 Supervised Exercise Therapy (SET)

Arguably the most important intervention in terms of overall benefit for the patient may be supervised exercise therapy. It has been found to promote angiogenesis [25], improve endothelial function [26], and increase muscle strength [27]. A meta-analysis has demonstrated an improvement of 50–200% in walking ability (4.5 min increase in mean maximal walking time, increase in pain-free walking of 82 m, increase in maximal walking distance of 109 m at 2 years) [18]. Supervised exercise therapy is defined as including the following: at least three times per week, at least 30 min per session, and at least 12 weeks in total duration and interval training with moderate claudication at rest point.

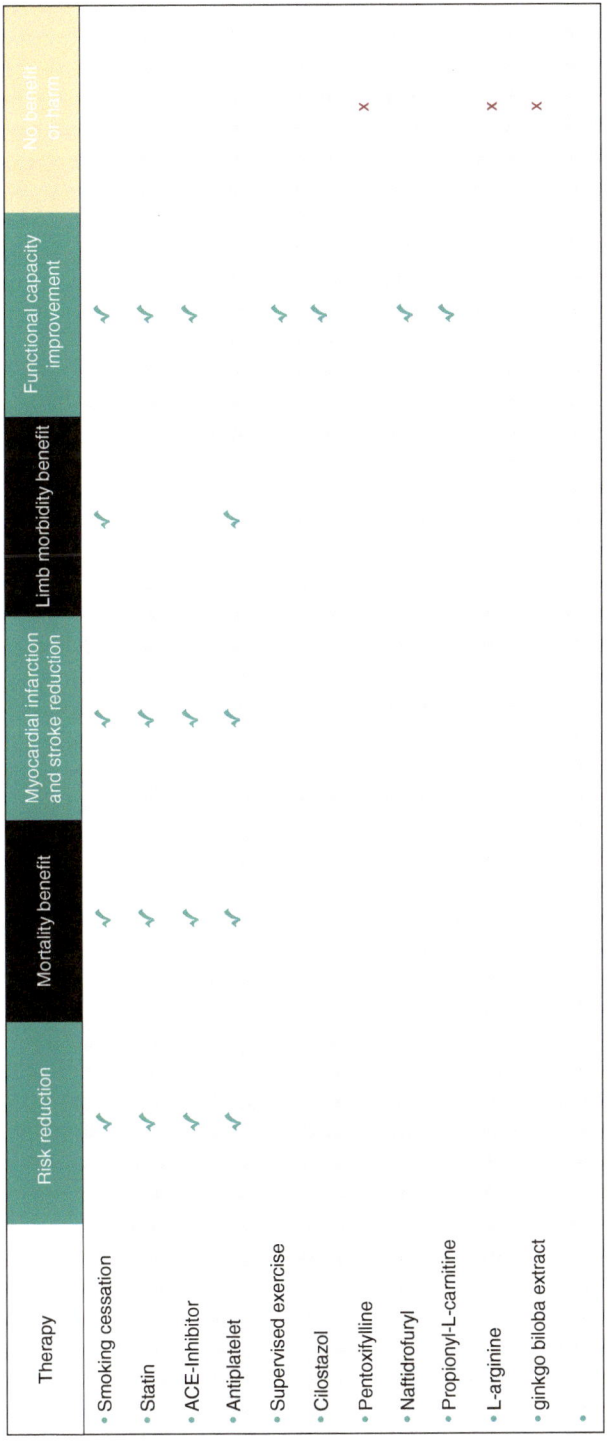

Therapy	Risk reduction	Mortality benefit	Myocardial infarction and stroke reduction	Limb morbidity benefit	Functional capacity improvement	No benefit or harm
• Smoking cessation	✓	✓	✓		✓	
• Statin	✓	✓	✓	✓	✓	
• ACE-Inhibitor	✓	✓	✓		✓	
• Antiplatelet	✓	✓	✓	✓		
• Supervised exercise					✓	
• Cilostazol					✓	
• Pentoxifylline					✓	✗
• Naftidrofuryl					✓	
• Propionyl-L-carnitine					✓	
• L-arginine						✗
• ginkgo biloba extract						✗

Fig. 1.1 Peripheral arterial disease therapeutics

1.4.2   Cilostazol

Cilostazol is a unique drug in that it inhibits phosphodiesterase 3 leading to an increase in cyclic adenosine monophosphate and subsequent arterial smooth muscle dilation via increased levels of nitrogen oxide. Though cilostazol has failed to demonstrate a mortality benefit, it has been found to be useful in improving functional capacity; it has been shown to result in a twofold improvement in maximal walking distance (absolute improvement of 42 m). Additionally, for the patients undergoing endovascular interventions, cilostazol has been shown to be useful in reducing restonsis [28, 29].

1.5   Therapeutics: Investigational, Failed, and Other Therapies

Various therapeutics have been trialed in the treatment of PAD to no avail. Pentoxifylline is a medication with numerous proposed mechanisms of action including inhibition of platelet aggregation and lowering of plasma fibrinogen levels. Though it has been in use for many years, there is no evidence that it is any more effective than placebo [30]. Naftidrofuryl is a medication which purportedly acts as a vasodilator as well as an enhancer of cellular oxidative capacity. Though not available in the United States of America, it has been approved for use in the European Union since 1972. Meta-analyses have both demonstrated a similar benefit as cilostazol with naftidrofuryl in regard to functional capacity improvement when compared to pentoxifylline [31]. Propionyl-L-carnitine is a key amino acid involved in the pathway of free fatty acid and glucose oxidation, both of which are altered in patients with PAD. In animal models a reduction in oxidative stress has been seen with carnitine supplementation [32]. In a meta-analysis of human subjects, carnitine therapy, a trend toward functional benefit with improvements in maximum walking, was seen with the greatest benefit in those patients with severe claudication [33]. L-Arginine is another amino acid that has been hypothesized to be of benefit as it is a precursor to nitric oxide a potent vasodilator. In the NO-PAIN study, 3 g of daily oral supplementation with L-arginine over a 6-month period in patients with PAD resulted in a statistically significant lower improvement in functional capacity as compared to placebo [34]. As such L-arginine is felt to be of no benefit and may even be harmful to patients when taken chronically. Similarly, *Ginkgo biloba* extract, a vasoactive agent, has been studied in numerous small trials for patients with PAD. A recent Cochrane meta-analysis demonstrated no clinically significant benefit of *Ginkgo biloba* extract supplementation in patients with PAD [35].

1.6   Conclusion

Peripheral arterial disease is a common and often underdiagnosed and undertreated vascular condition. Control of risk factors, especially smoking cessation, is the mainstay of therapy for the reduction of cardiovascular morbidity and mortality. The addition of antiplatelet therapies as well as supervised exercise therapy among other therapeutics is often of benefit as well for functional improvement in walking capacity.

References

1. Pasternak RC et al. Atherosclerotic vascular disease conference: writing group I: epidemiology. Circulation. 2004;109(21):2605–12.
2. Krupski WC. The peripheral vascular consequences of smoking. Ann Vasc Surg. 1991;5(3):291–304.
3. Bartholomew JR, Olin JW. Pathophysiology of peripheral arterial disease and risk factors for its development. Cleve Clin J Med. 2006;73(Suppl 4):S8–14.
4. He Y et al. Passive smoking and risk of peripheral arterial disease and ischemic stroke in Chinese women who never smoked. Circulation. 2008;118(15):1535–40.
5. Grana R, Benowitz N, Glantz SA. E-cigarettes: a scientific review. Circulation. 2014;129(19):1972–86.
6. Valentine RJ et al. Lp(a) lipoprotein is an independent, discriminating risk factor for premature peripheral atherosclerosis among white men. Arch Intern Med. 1994;154(7):801–6.
7. Kannel WB, McGee DL. Update on some epidemiologic features of intermittent claudication: the Framingham Study. J Am Geriatr Soc. 1985;33(1):13–8.
8. Newman AB et al. Ankle-arm index as a marker of atherosclerosis in the Cardiovascular Health Study. Cardiovascular Heart Study (CHS) Collaborative Research Group. Circulation. 1993;88(3):837–45.
9. Selvin E et al. Meta-analysis: glycosylated hemoglobin and cardiovascular disease in diabetes mellitus. Ann Intern Med. 2004;141(6):421–31.
10. Jude EB et al. Peripheral arterial disease in diabetic and nondiabetic patients: a comparison of severity and outcome. Diabetes Care. 2001;24(8):1433–7.
11. Quick CR, Cotton LT. The measured effect of stopping smoking on intermittent claudication. Br J Surg. 1982;69(Suppl):S24–6.
12. Jonason T, Bergstrom R. Cessation of smoking in patients with intermittent claudication. Effects on the risk of peripheral vascular complications, myocardial infarction and mortality. Acta Med Scand. 1987;221(3):253–60.
13. Clinical Practice Guideline Treating Tobacco Use and Dependence 2008 Update Panel, Liaisons, and Staff. A clinical practice guideline for treating tobacco use and dependence: 2008 update. A U.S. Public Health Service report. Am J Prev Med. 2008;35(2):158–76.
14. Silagy C et al. Nicotine replacement therapy for smoking cessation. Cochrane Database Syst Rev. 2004;(3):CD000146.
15. Gonzales D et al. Varenicline, an alpha4beta2 nicotinic acetylcholine receptor partial agonist, vs sustained-release bupropion and placebo for smoking cessation: a randomized controlled trial. JAMA. 2006;296(1):47–55.
16. Jorenby DE et al. A controlled trial of sustained-release bupropion, a nicotine patch, or both for smoking cessation. N Engl J Med. 1999;340(9):685–91.

17. Rooke TW et al. Management of patients with peripheral artery disease (compilation of 2005 and 2011 ACCF/AHA Guideline Recommendations): a report of the American College of Cardiology Foundation/American Heart Association Task Force on Practice Guidelines. J Am Coll Cardiol. 2013;61(14):1555–70.
18. Lane R et al. Exercise for intermittent claudication. Cochrane Database Syst Rev. 2014;(7):CD000990.
19. Yusuf S et al. Effects of an angiotensin-converting-enzyme inhibitor, ramipril, on cardiovascular events in high-risk patients. The Heart Outcomes Prevention Evaluation Study Investigators. N Engl J Med. 2000;342(3):145–53.
20. Ahimastos AA et al. Effect of ramipril on walking times and quality of life among patients with peripheral artery disease and intermittent claudication: a randomized controlled trial. JAMA. 2013;309(5):453–60.
21. Antithrombotic Trialists' Collaboration. Collaborative meta-analysis of randomised trials of antiplatelet therapy for prevention of death, myocardial infarction, and stroke in high risk patients. BMJ. 2002;324(7329):71–86.
22. Goldhaber SZ et al. Low-dose aspirin and subsequent peripheral arterial surgery in the Physicians' Health Study. Lancet. 1992;340(8812):143–5.
23. Committee CS. A randomised, blinded, trial of clopidogrel versus aspirin in patients at risk of ischaemic events (CAPRIE). CAPRIE Steering Committee. Lancet. 1996;348(9038):1329–39.
24. Bhatt DL et al. Patients with prior myocardial infarction, stroke, or symptomatic peripheral arterial disease in the CHARISMA trial. J Am Coll Cardiol. 2007;49(19):1982–8.
25. Gustafsson T, Kraus WE. Exercise-induced angiogenesis-related growth and transcription factors in skeletal muscle, and their modification in muscle pathology. Front Biosci. 2001;6:D75–89.
26. Brendle DC et al. Effects of exercise rehabilitation on endothelial reactivity in older patients with peripheral arterial disease. Am J Cardiol. 2001;87(3):324–9.
27. Hiatt WR et al. Effect of exercise training on skeletal muscle histology and metabolism in peripheral arterial disease. J Appl Physiol (1985). 1996;81(2):780–8.
28. Pande RL et al. A pooled analysis of the durability and predictors of treatment response of cilostazol in patients with intermittent claudication. Vasc Med. 2010;15(3):181–8.
29. Dawson DL et al. Cilostazol has beneficial effects in treatment of intermittent claudication: results from a multicenter, randomized, prospective, double-blind trial. Circulation. 1998;98(7):678–86.
30. Ernst E. Pentoxifylline for intermittent claudication. A critical review. Angiology. 1994;45(5):339–45.
31. Stevens JW et al. Systematic review of the efficacy of cilostazol, naftidrofuryl oxalate and pentoxifylline for the treatment of intermittent claudication. Br J Surg. 2012;99(12):1630–8.
32. Dutta A et al. L-carnitine supplementation attenuates intermittent hypoxia-induced oxidative stress and delays muscle fatigue in rats. Exp Physiol. 2008;93(10):1139–46.
33. Delaney CL et al. A systematic review to evaluate the effectiveness of carnitine supplementation in improving walking performance among individuals with intermittent claudication. Atherosclerosis. 2013;229(1):1–9.
34. Wilson AM et al. L-arginine supplementation in peripheral arterial disease: no benefit and possible harm. Circulation. 2007;116(2):188–95.
35. Nicolai SP et al. *Ginkgo biloba* for intermittent claudication. Cochrane Database Syst Rev. 2013;6:CD006888.

Chapter 2
Endovascular Treatment of Iliac Artery Chronic Total Occlusions

Kalkidan Bishu and Ehrin J. Armstrong

2.1 Introduction

Approximately 8.5 million American adults are affected by peripheral artery disease (PAD). The iliac arteries and infrarenal aorta are among the arterial circulations most commonly affected by atherosclerotic chronic total occlusion (CTO) and constitute approximately one third of cases of PAD. Percutaneous angioplasty for iliac CTO was first described by Tegtmeyer et al. in 1979 in a 55-year-old diabetic woman with nonhealing foot ulcers in association with a CTO of the right common iliac artery (CIA) [1]. While surgical bypass can be performed with high long-term patency for aortoiliac PAD, endovascular interventions are increasingly being used to treat disabling claudication in such patients [2]. Surgical bypass options vary based on the specific anatomy, but include aortofemoral or aorta bi-femoral bypass, iliofemoral bypass, femoral-femoral bypass, and aortoiliac endarterectomy. Surgical bypass is associated with satisfactory improvement in symptoms and long-term patency rates, but such operations may incur significant operative morbidity and mortality. Thus endovascular aortoiliac interventions are often considered as a first-line treatment strategy for symptomatic patients with aortoiliac disease [2, 3].

The Trans-Atlantic Inter-Society Consensus (TASC) II document provides a classification of aortoiliac lesions according to the level of complexity (types A, B, C, and D) that can be used to guide the revascularization approach (Fig. 2.1) [4].

Conflict of Interest (or Disclosures) EJA is a consultant for Abbott Vascular, Medtronic, Merck, Pfizer, and Spectranetics.

K. Bishu, MD, MS • E.J. Armstrong, MD, MSc, MAS (✉)
Division of Cardiology, University of Colorado, Aurora, CO, USA

Denver VA Medical Center, 1055 Clermont Street, Denver, CO 80220, USA
e-mail: Ehrin.armstrong@gmail.com

© Springer Science+Business Media Singapore 2017
S. Banerjee (ed.), *Practical Approach to Peripheral Arterial Chronic Total Occlusions*, DOI 10.1007/978-981-10-3053-6_2

Type A lesions

• Unilateral or bilateral stenoses of CIA
• Unilateral or bilateral single short (≤3 cm) stenosis of EIA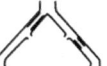

Type B lesions

• Short (≤3cm) stenosis of infrarenal aorta
• Unilateral CIA occlusion
• Single or multiple stenosis totaling 3–10 cm involving the
  EIA not extending into the CFA
• Unilateral EIA occlusion not involving the origins of
  internal iliac or CFA

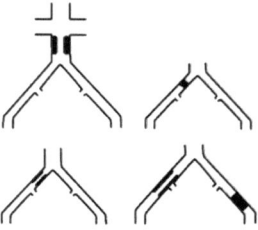

Type C lesions

• Bilateral CIA occlusions
• Bilateral EIA stenosis 3–10 cm long not extending into
  the CFA
• Unilateral EIA stenosis extending into the CFA
• Unilateral EIA occlusion that involves the origins of
  internal iliac and/or CFA
• Heavily calcified unilateral EIA occlusion with or without
  involvement of origins of internal iliac and/or CFA

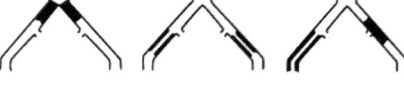

Type D lesions

• Infra-renal aortoiliac occlusion
• Diffuse disease involving the aorta and both iliac arteries
  requiring treatment
• Diffuse multiple stenoses involving the unilateral CIA,
  EIA, and CFA
• Unilateral occlusions of both CIA and EIA
• Bilateral occlusions of EIA
• Iliac stenoses in patients with AAA requiring treatment
  and not amenable to endograft placement or other
  lesions requiring open aortic or iliac surgery

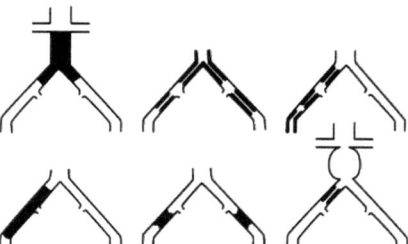

Fig. 2.1 TASC II classification of aortoiliac peripheral arterial disease. *CIA* common iliac artery, *EIA* external iliac artery, *CFA* common femoral artery, *AAA* abdominal aortic aneurysm (Reproduced with permission from Norgren et al. [4])

Type A lesions are the least complex focal stenoses of the CIA or the external iliac artery (EIA). Type B lesions are unilateral CIA or EIA occlusions (not involving the common femoral artery (CFA) or internal iliac artery (IIA) origins). Type C lesions are bilateral CIA occlusions, unilateral EIA occlusions that are heavily calcified or involve the CFA or IIA origins. Type D occlusions include aortoiliac occlusion, unilateral occlusions of the CIA and EIA, and bilateral EIA occlusions. While the TASC documents recommended endovascular treatment for type B occlusions and surgical bypass for type C and type D lesions, with increasing operator experience, type C and D lesions are increasingly being treated via an endovascular approach [5]. In addition, procedural success rate does not appear to be a function of the TASC II classification (which is primarily defined by anatomic involvement) and may instead be related to underlying characteristics of the occluded segment (e.g., calcification, ease of reentry, etc.).

2.2 Outcomes After Endovascular Treatment of Iliac CTOs

Endovascular recanalization assisted with stenting is increasingly being performed in the treatment of iliac CTOs with satisfactory long-term patency rates. Stenting is the primary strategy in the endovascular treatment of iliac occlusions and is associated with high long-term patency rates compared to angioplasty alone [6]. In a meta-analysis of 1300 patients with iliac disease treated with angioplasty or angioplasty with stenting, among patients with stenosis as well as occlusions, patency rates at 4 years were superior for stenting compared to angioplasty alone (61% vs. 54% for chronic limb ischemia patients with iliac CTOs and 53% vs. 44% for claudicants with iliac CTOs) [6].

Most other data regarding long-term outcomes of iliac CTOs treated with stenting are limited to observational studies of one or two centers. Scheinert et al. treated 212 patients with unilateral iliac CTOs via an endovascular approach with excimer laser-assisted recanalization and stent implantation [7]. The authors reported an 84% primary patency rate at 1 year. Contralateral crossover antegrade crossing of the lesion was accomplished in 91%, whereas in the remaining 9% an ipsilateral retrograde approach was used. Similarly, Carnevale et al. treated 69 iliac CTOs with a 97% technical success rate [8]. The primary patency at 1 year was 91%. Leville et al. treated 89 patients with iliac CTOs with a 91% procedural success rate. Three-year primary patency was 76%. The prevalence of TASC B, C, and D lesions was 25%, 34%, and 42%, respectively. Technical success rates were similar at 95%, 94%, and 86% in the different TASC groups, respectively [9].

In a larger observational study, Ozkan et al. treated 127 limbs in 118 patients with iliac CTOs. Lesions were in the common iliac artery, external iliac artery, and combined common and external iliac arteries in 53%, 28%, and 19% of patients, respectively [10]. Seven percent of patients had bilateral common iliac artery (CIA) occlusions, most of whom had total aortoiliac occlusions. Recanalization was attempted from the ipsilateral retrograde approach first, which was successful in 50% of cases. In the case of failed ipsilateral approach, a contralateral crossover antegrade approach was attempted which was subsequently successful in 90% of cases. Primary patency at 5 years was 63%.

Multiple other studies have suggested that the TASC II classification of iliac CTOs may not be associated with procedural success or long-term patency. Chen et al. treated 120 patients with iliac CTOs with successful recanalization in 101 CTOs. 39%, 27%, and 35% of lesions were TASC II types B, C, and D, respectively. A reentry device (Pioneer or Outback) was required in 14% of lesions that were successfully revascularized. The primary patency at 1 year was 86% [10]. Dattilo et al. performed 63 iliac CTO endovascular interventions with a procedural success rate of 97%. 59%, 7%, and 37% of lesions were TASC II types B, C, and D, respectively [5]. Technical success rates were not different in the different TASC II subtypes. Papakostas et al. treated iliac CTOs in 56 limbs in 48 patients by the endovascular approach with stent implantation with a 91% procedural success rate. 30%, 32%, and 38% of lesions were TASC II types B, C, and D, respectively. Primary patency (peak systolic velocity of <2.5% on arterial duplex US) at 3 years was 91%. TASC II type was not associated with procedural success or patency [11].

In summary, current observational studies have demonstrated that iliac artery CTOs can be treated via endovascular techniques with success rates exceeding 90% in most cases. The long-term patency of iliac artery CTOs is also high after successful endovascular treatment, suggesting that endovascular treatment of iliac artery CTOs is a reasonable first-line treatment strategy for most symptomatic iliac artery CTOs.

2.3 Treatment Strategies and Illustrative Cases

The approach to iliac CTO endovascular recanalization primarily depends on the anatomic location of the occlusion. This section provides a general overview for treatment of iliac artery CTOs, followed by illustrative cases that demonstrate the technical approach to treatment of specific anatomic subgroups.

2.3.1 Overall Approach and Treatment Strategy

Endovascular treatment of iliac artery CTOs should be based on detailed pre-procedure planning in order to determine the optimal treatment approach and maximize the chances of technical success. In cases where an iliac artery CTO is suspected, pre-procedural CTA imaging can be invaluable in providing specific anatomic detail including the presence and amount of vessel calcification, the location of occlusion and site of reconstitution, and the location of collateral vessels.

Multiple sites of arterial access may be necessary for successful treatment of iliac artery CTOs. Whenever possible, a 7 French sheath should be employed; the larger sheath size makes it possible to deliver covered stents and/or a larger occlusion balloon in the case of iliac artery perforation. The most frequent access involves bilateral common femoral artery access, in order to provide adequate vessel imaging from above and multiple treatment options, including combined antegrade/retrograde crossing in case of challenging lesion crossing. Brachial access may provide additional backup support for challenging lesions, especially ostial or proximal occlusions of the common iliac artery. In such cases, left brachial access should be obtained, and a 90 cm shuttle sheath used to maximize backup support [12]. Radial access may also be useful for aortoiliac imaging or for treatment of proximal common iliac artery disease [13]. However, the shaft length of most endovascular devices makes treatment of more distal external iliac lesions difficult from a radial approach. Rarely, popliteal or pedal access may be necessary for successful treatment of an iliac artery CTO, but should be reserved for cases where there is concomitant common femoral artery disease that may need to be treated from a retrograde approach in order to preserve the bifurcation of the profunda femoris with the superficial femoral artery.

The optimal approach for crossing an iliac artery CTO remains uncertain. Retrograde crossing from ipsilateral common femoral artery access has the advantage of treating from the same side, thereby avoiding the need for a crossover sheath. However, imaging from a retrograde sheath is often suboptimal, and contralateral access may be required regardless to image the proximal lesion cap. Antegrade access may have a higher success rate for crossing of the occlusion, but subsequent treatment usually requires wire externalization, which increases the overall complexity of the procedure. If one wire crossing strategy is not successful, it is reasonable to switch strategies and attempt a "true lumen" crossing from the other direction prior to using dedicated reentry techniques. In some cases, wire advancement may be necessary from both directions simultaneously, followed by a "CART" or "reverse CART" technique to reconcile the subintimal space and cross the cap into the true lumen [14].

No specific data exists on the optimal stent type for treatment of iliac CTOs. Most operators choose a strategy of balloon expandable stents for treatment of common iliac artery disease due to the more predictable deployment of such stents, and a self-expanding stent for treatment of external iliac artery disease, due to the increased conformability of these stents in the tortuous external iliac artery. The COBEST trial did demonstrate superior patency of covered balloon expandable stents in the treatment of TASC C and TASC D lesions, suggesting that this stent type may have some relative benefit in the treatment of complex iliac artery CTOs [15].

2.3.2   Ostial Common Iliac or Aortic Bifurcation

Treatment of ostial CIA occlusion or aortic bifurcation disease involving the bilateral common iliac ostia can most often be accomplished using bilateral retrograde common femoral artery (CFA) access and kissing angioplasty/stenting. Crossing the lesion may be attempted from the retrograde approach initially. Such an approach is associated with 50% success rate [10]. If this approach fails, contralateral crossover antegrade approach is usually successful in crossing the lesion, with a reported 90% success rate based on limited data. Ultrasound guidance or roadmaps are helpful in accessing the patency of the CFA distal to a CIA occlusion, which can determine the use of a short brite tip sheath for distal access. A 7F sheath is required usually due to the caliber of stents required to treat CIA disease, especially if balloon expandable covered stents are used. The stents should be extended approximately 5 mm into the distal abdominal aorta, but the extent of coverage depends on the presence of distal abdominal aorta disease and the angulation of the bifurcation.

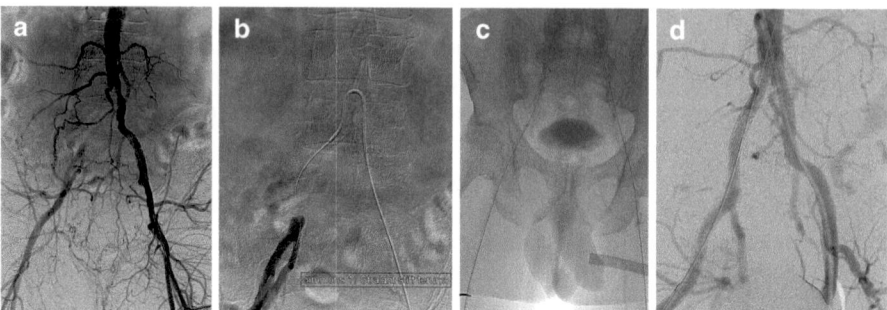

Fig. 2.2 Digital subtraction aortoiliac angiography showing right CIA occlusion involving the ostium (**a**). Lesion crossed using a 0.035″ straight stiff Glidewire supported by a Simmons 1 catheter (**b**). The wire was exteriorized through the right CFA sheath (**c**). Atrium iCAST stents deployed in kissing stent fashion at bilateral iliac artery origins into the distal abdominal aorta (**d**)

Such an approach will usually prohibit contralateral crossover during subsequent procedures, especially if the stents are extended into the distal aorta. When the common iliac branches are larger in caliber and the distal abdominal aorta may not accommodate the two stents protruding into its lumen, a self-expanding stent may be used. In rare cases, self-expanding covered iliac stent grafts (which are typically used for endovascular aortic repair) may be necessary to accommodate ectatic iliac arteries.

Illustrative cases using an endovascular approach to treat ostial CIA disease are described below:

Case 1. A 65-year-old male with Rutherford Class III right lower extremity claudication and an ostial right CIA occlusion (Fig. 2.2a) was brought to the cardiac catheterization laboratory. 7F bilateral CFA access was obtained using ultrasound guidance and a micropuncture technique. An initial attempt at crossing the occlusion from the right ipsilateral retrograde direction with a 0.035″ straight stiff Glidewire was unsuccessful. A contralateral antegrade approach was successful in crossing the lesion using a 0.035″ straight stiff Glidewire supported by a Simmons 1 catheter (Fig. 2.2a). The wire was exteriorized through the right CFA sheath (Fig. 2.2c) followed by angioplasty and placement of balloon expandable covered stents in kissing stent fashion at the bilateral common iliac artery origins into the distal abdominal aorta (Fig. 2.2d).

Case 2. A 68-year-old male presented with Rutherford Class III bilateral lower extremity claudication. There was a CTO of the left CIA including the ostium and severe proximal stenosis of the right CIA (Fig. 2.3a). 7F bilateral CFA access was obtained using ultrasound guidance and a micropuncture technique. The left CIA occlusion was crossed using a 0.035″ straight stiff Glidewire from the ipsilateral retrograde approach supported by a Navicross catheter (Fig. 2.3b, c). Kissing balloon angioplasty was performed followed by kissing stents placed in the bilateral common iliac arteries proximally extending into the distal abdominal aorta using balloon expandable covered stents (Fig. 2.3d).

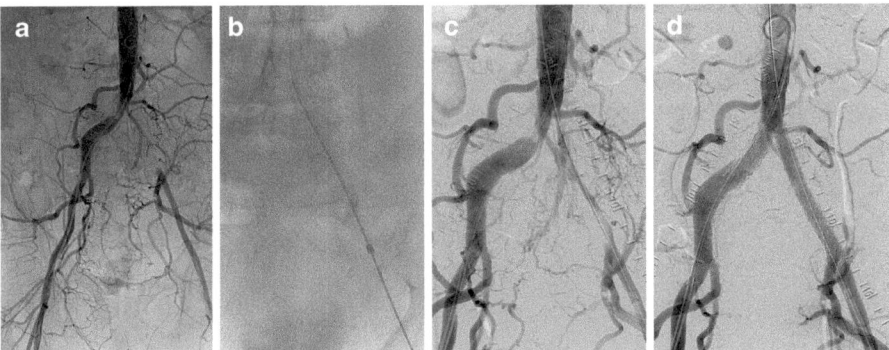

Fig. 2.3 Digital subtraction aortoiliac angiography showing left CIA occlusion involving the ostium (**a**). The left CIA occlusion was crossed using a 0.035″ straight stiff Glidewire from the ipsilateral retrograde approach supported by a Navicross catheter (**b, c**). Kissing stents were placed in bilateral common iliac arteries proximally extending into the distal abdominal aorta using Atrium iCAST balloon covered expandable stents (**d**)

The strategy of using aortoiliac kissing stents has been shown to maintain long-term patency in multiple studies. Mendelsohn et al. treated 20 patients with kissing iliac stents for aortoiliac artery disease involving both ($n = 15$) common iliac artery origins and complex unilateral iliac artery ostial disease [16]. Scheinert et al. treated 48 patients with aortoiliac bifurcation disease (including 22 with unilateral occlusion and contralateral stenosis and one patient with bilateral iliac occlusion) with excimer laser-assisted recanalization and kissing stent placement [17]. The primary angiographic patency at 2 years was 87%. Yilmaz et al. treated 68 patients with aortoiliac disease (including 26 patients with unilateral CIA occlusion and contralateral stenosis) with kissing stents [18]. The primary patency at 1 year was 76%. Self-expanding stents were used in 76%, and balloon expandable stents were used in 24% of patients. Mohamed et al. treated 24 patients with aortoiliac disease with kissing stents and reported a 1-year primary rate of 81% [19]. Predominantly self-expanding stents were used. Bjorses et al. reviewed the use of kissing stents in 173 patients with aortoiliac occlusive disease and reported a 1-year primary patency rate of 97% [20]. Fifty-one percent of patients received self-expanding stents, 30% received balloon expandable stents, 13% received a combination of self-expanding and balloon expandable stents, whereas 6% of patients received covered stents. Haulon et al. reported the results of 106 patients treated with aortoiliac kissing stents with a primary 1-year patency rate of 79% [21]. Self-expanding stents were used in 59% of cases, whereas balloon expandable stents were used in 41% of cases. Some limited data also suggests that covered balloon expandable stents may be superior to bare metal balloon expandable stents at the aortic bifurcation. Sabri et al. treated 26 patients with aortoiliac disease with covered balloon expandable stents and 28 patients with bare metal balloon expandable stents in a kissing stent fashion and noted superior long-term patency with the covered stents (92% vs. 78% 1-year patency rate) [22].

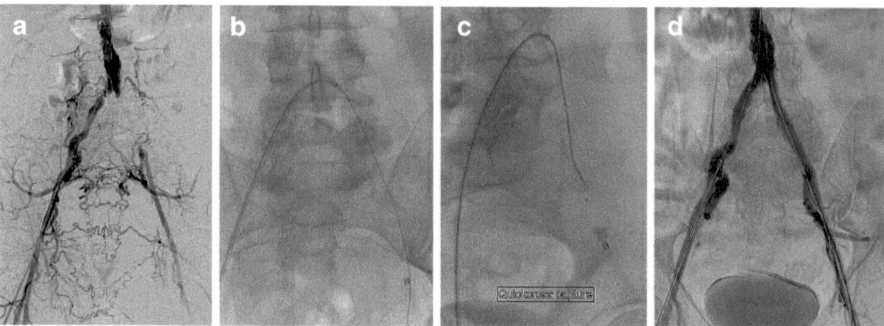

Fig. 2.4 Digital subtraction aortoiliac angiography showing left CIA occlusion involving the ostium (**a**). Contralateral right CFA sheath was exchanged for a Morph AccessPro steerable sheath which was advanced to the distal abdominal aorta and used to provide support for crossing the left CIA lesion with a straight stiff 0.035″ Glidewire from the contralateral crossover retrograde approach (**b**). A Quick-Cross Capture catheter was advanced in the left CFA sheath and advanced to the left EIA where the wire used to cross the occlusion from the retrograde approach was captured and exteriorized into the ipsilateral sheath (**c**). iCAST covered balloon expandable stents were delivered from the ipsilateral approach into bilateral proximal common iliac arteries and deployed (**d**)

Case 3. A 68-year-old male with severe left lower extremity claudication was found to have a left proximal common iliac CTO involving the ostium (Fig. 2.4a). 7F bilateral CFA access was obtained. After an initial unsuccessful attempt at crossing the lesion from the ipsilateral retrograde approach, the contralateral right CFA sheath was exchanged for a Morph AccessPro steerable sheath, which was advanced to the distal abdominal aorta and used to provide support for crossing the left CIA lesion with a straight stiff 0.035″ Glidewire from the contralateral crossover retrograde approach (Fig. 2.4b). A Quick-Cross Capture catheter was advanced in the left CFA sheath and advanced to the left external iliac artery (EIA) where the wire that had been used to cross the occlusion from the retrograde approach was captured and exteriorized into the ipsilateral sheath (Fig. 2.4c). iCAST covered balloon expandable stents were delivered from the ipsilateral approach into bilateral proximal common iliac arteries and deployed (Fig. 2.4d).

2.3.3 Non-ostial Common Iliac Artery and Proximal External Iliac Artery CTOs

Non-ostial common iliac artery and proximal external iliac artery CTOs can be treated from an ipsilateral CFA retrograde or a contralateral antegrade approach. Common iliac artery CTOs with a proximal stump can also be treated from either the retrograde or the antegrade approach using crossover contralateral access or brachial access.

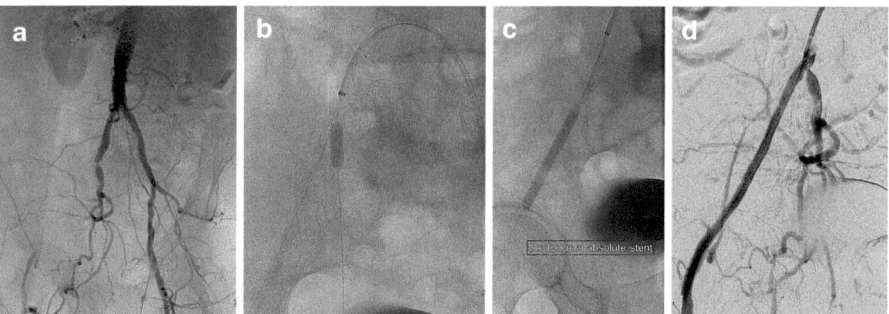

Fig. 2.5 Digital subtraction angiography with landmarking demonstrated a CTO of the right external iliac artery (**a**). The occlusion is in the proximal external iliac artery, and there is also significant stenosis at the origin of the internal iliac artery. A crossover sheath was advanced to the right common iliac artery, and a straight stiff 0.035″ Glidewire was used to cross the occlusion. Due to significant stenosis at the ostium of the internal iliac artery, a wire was also passed into this vessel, and balloon angioplasty was performed (**b**). A self-expanding stent was placed in the right external iliac artery (**c**). Final angiography revealed patency of the right internal iliac artery and external iliac artery (**d**)

Case 4. A 54-year-old man with a history of Rutherford III right lower extremity claudication underwent lower extremity angiography, which revealed an occluded right external iliac artery just distal to the origin of the right internal iliac artery (Fig. 2.5a). The lesion was approached from a contralateral antegrade approach, and the occlusion was successfully crossed using a straight stiff 0.035″ Glidewire into the true lumen of the distal external iliac artery. Because of the high-grade disease at the origin of the right internal iliac artery, a 0.014″ wire was advanced into the internal iliac artery, and balloon angioplasty was performed at the ostium of the internal iliac artery (Fig. 2.5b). A self-expanding stent was then placed along the length of the right external iliac artery (Fig. 2.5c), with excellent angiographic result (Fig. 2.5d).

2.3.4   Distal External Iliac Artery CTOs

Distal external iliac artery lesions are ideally treated using a contralateral crossover approach, due to the potential difficulty in gaining arterial access in the ipsilateral common femoral artery and attendant lack of sheath support. Balloon expandable stents may be used if in close proximity to the hip joint due to the concern regarding failure of self-expanding stents in this location. A contralateral crossover sheath can be placed with its tip in the CIA and used to cross the occlusion and perform angioplasty and stenting from the antegrade approach.

An illustrative case of the endovascular treatment of an external iliac CTO is described below.

Case 5. A 72-year-old male with Rutherford Class III right lower extremity claudication and a history of prior left EIA stenting was brought to the catheterization

laboratory. There was a chronic occlusion of the length of the external iliac artery
(Fig. 2.6a). A 6F Morph AccessPro steerable sheath was advanced in the left CFA
and directed into the right CIA. A 0.035″ support wire was advanced into the right
internal iliac artery for advancement of a crossover sheath into the right CIA (Fig.
2.6b). A 0.035″ stiff Glidewire was directed into the EIA on the right but remained
in the subintimal space. Right dorsalis pedis access was obtained, and a Prowater
0.14″ wire was advanced retrograde into the right EIA but remained in the subintimal

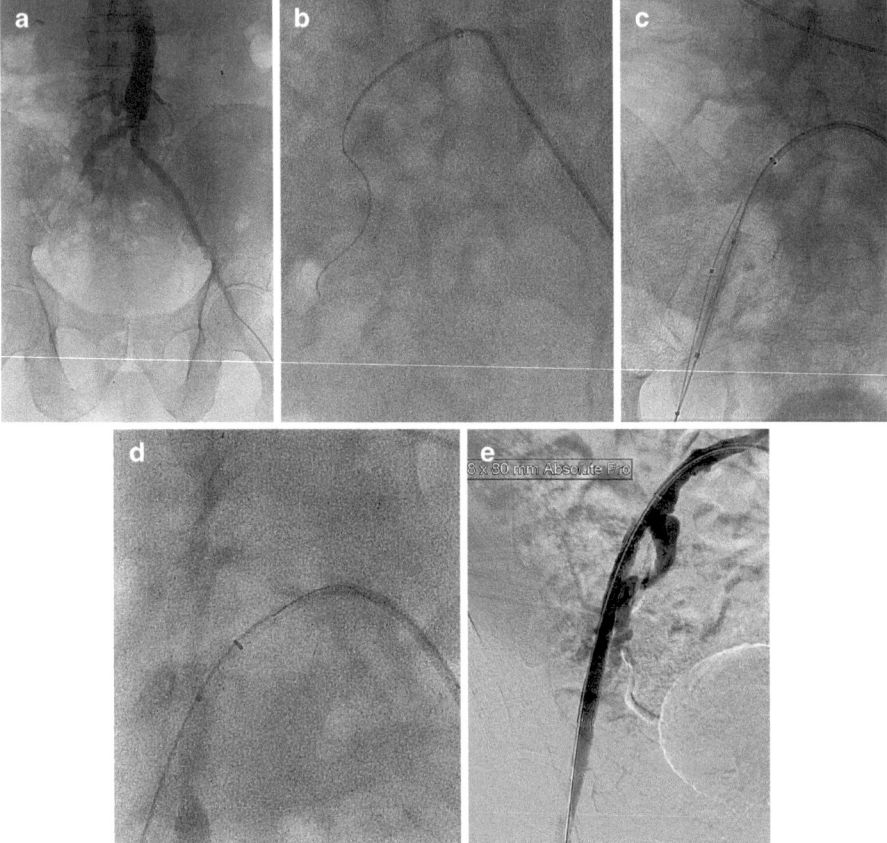

Fig. 2.6 Digital subtraction angiography showing CTO of the right external iliac artery (**a**).
Following placement of a 6F Morph AccessPro steerable sheath was in the left CFA and directed
into the right CIA, and 0.035 support wire was advanced to the right internal iliac artery for
advancement of a crossover sheath into the right CIA (**b**). Reverse-controlled antegrade and retrograde subintimal tracking (CART) technique. A 0.035″ wire in the subintimal space from the
crossover antegrade approach with a Charger balloon and a 0.014″ guide wire placed retrograde in
the subintimal space from the ipsilateral DP (**c**). The retrograde advanced Probate wire used to
reenter the luminal space and externalized through the cross over sheath in the left CFA (**d**). An 8
× 80 Absolute Pro self-expanding stent advanced antegrade from the contralateral approach and
deployed along the length of the EIA on the right (**e**)

space. A 6.0 × 40 mm Charger balloon was advanced over the 0.035 wire that was advanced antegrade in the subintimal space in the right EIA and inflated in the subintimal space to create a communication with the separate subintimal space created by the retrograde wire within the occlusion of the right EIA. The retrograde Prowater wire was used to reenter the luminal space and directed into the right EIA and CIA and was externalized through the sheath in the left CFA (Fig. 2.6d). The wire was exchanged for a 0.035″ guide wire over which angioplasty was performed from the retrograde approach. An 8 × 80 mm Absolute Pro self-expanding stent was advanced from the contralateral approach and deployed along the length of the EIA on the right (Fig. 2.6e).

The successful use of the controlled antegrade and retrograde subintimal tracking (CART) technique, initially described to facilitate recanalization of coronary CTOs, has been successfully used in the treatment of EIA occlusion in the past [14]. In this case we describe the use of reverse CART technique in which the occlusion is crossed from a retrograde wire in the subintimal space. Intravascular ultrasound-guided true lumen reentry devices have also been used for recanalization of iliac artery occlusion [23]. A 100% technical success rate was reported in a series of 11 patients (seven, one, and three patients had unilateral CIA, EIA, and combined CIA/EIA occlusions). The Pioneer reentry catheter was used in that study, although the Outback catheter can also be used for successful reentry of iliac artery CTOs [10].

2.4 Conclusions

Iliac artery chronic occlusions are a source of increased morbidity among patients with PAD. While surgical bypass has a high long-term patency, it is associated with significant morbidity. Recent advances in techniques and equipment used for endovascular recanalization have made the endovascular approach a plausible option for the initial treatment of patients with iliac CTOs, with a procedural success rate exceeding 90%. Future research should better define the optimal initial crossing strategy in order to maximize the chances of expedient occlusion crossing. Additional data regarding the outcomes of different stent types will also be helpful in defining the optimal endovascular treatment of iliac artery CTOs.

References

1. Tegtmeyer CJ, Moore TS, Chandler JG, Wellons HA, Rudolf LE. Percutaneous transluminal dilatation of a complete block in the right iliac artery. AJR Am J Roentgenol. 1979;133:532–5.
2. Hirsch AT, Haskal ZJ, Hertzer NR, Bakal CW, Creager MA, Halperin JL, Hiratzka LF, Murphy WRC, Olin JW, Puschett JB, Rosenfield KA, Sacks D, Stanley JC, Taylor LM, White CJ, White J, White RA, Antman EM, Smith SC, Adams CD, Anderson JL, Faxon DP, Fuster V, Gibbons RJ, Hunt SA, Jacobs AK, Nishimura R, Ornato JP, Page RL, Riegel B, American

Association for Vascular Surgery, Society for Vascular Surgery, Society for Cardiovascular Angiography and Interventions, Society for Vascular Medicine and Biology, Society of Interventional Radiology, ACC/AHA Task Force on Practice Guidelines Writing Committee to Develop Guidelines for the Management of Patients With Peripheral Arterial Disease, American Association of Cardiovascular and Pulmonary Rehabilitation, National Heart Lung and Blood Institute, Society for Vascular Nursing, TransAtlantic Inter-Society Consensus, Vascular Disease Foundation. ACC/AHA 2005 practice guidelines for the management of patients with peripheral arterial disease (lower extremity, renal, mesenteric, and abdominal aortic): a collaborative report from the American Association for Vascular Surgery/Society for Vascular Surgery, Society for Cardiovascular Angiography and Interventions, Society for Vascular Medicine and Biology, Society of Interventional Radiology, and the ACC/AHA Task Force on Practice Guidelines (Writing Committee to Develop Guidelines for the Management of Patients With Peripheral Arterial Disease): endorsed by the American Association of Cardiovascular and Pulmonary Rehabilitation; National Heart, Lung, and Blood Institute; Society for Vascular Nursing; TransAtlantic Inter-Society Consensus; and Vascular Disease Foundation. J Am Coll Cardiol. 2006;113:e463–654.

3. Klein AJ, Feldman DN, Aronow HD, Gray BH, Gupta K, Gigliotti OS, Jaff MR, Bersin RM, White CJ, Peripheral Vascular Disease Committee for the Society for Cardiovascular Angiography and Interventions. SCAI expert consensus statement for aorto-iliac arterial intervention appropriate use. Cathet Cardiovasc Interv. 2014;84:520–8.

4. Norgren L, Hiatt WR, Dormandy JA, Nehler MR, Harris KA, Fowkes FGR, TASC II Working Group. Inter-Society Consensus for the Management of Peripheral Arterial Disease (TASC II). J Vasc Surg. 2007;45:S5–67.

5. Dattilo PB, Tsai TT, Garcia JA, Allshouse A, Casserly IP. Clinical outcomes with contemporary endovascular therapy of iliac artery occlusive disease. Catheter Cardiovasc Interv. 2012;80:644–54.

6. Bosch JL, Hunink MG. Meta-analysis of the results of percutaneous transluminal angioplasty and stent placement for aortoiliac occlusive disease. Radiology. 1997;204:87–96.

7. Scheinert D, Schröder M, Ludwig J, Bräunlich S, Möckel M, Flachskampf FA, Balzer JO, Biamino G. Stent-supported recanalization of chronic iliac artery occlusions. Am J Med. 2001;110:708–15.

8. Carnevale FC, De Blas M, Merino S, Egaña JM, Caldas JGMP. Percutaneous endovascular treatment of chronic iliac artery occlusion. Cardiovasc Intervent Radiol. 2004;27:447–52.

9. Leville CD, Kashyap VS, Clair DG, Bena JF, Lyden SP, Greenberg RK, O'Hara PJ, Sarac TP, Ouriel K. Endovascular management of iliac artery occlusions: extending treatment to TransAtlantic Inter-Society Consensus class C and D patients. J Vasc Surg. 2006;43:32–9.

10. Ozkan U, Oguzkurt L, Tercan F. Technique, complication, and long-term outcome for endovascular treatment of iliac artery occlusion. Cardiovasc Intervent Radiol. 2010;33:18–24.

11. Papakostas JC, Chatzigakis PK, Peroulis M, Avgos S, Kouvelos G, Lazaris A, Matsagkas MI. Endovascular treatment of chronic total occlusions of the iliac arteries. Early and mid-term results. Ann Vasc Surg. 2015;29:1508–15.

12. Millon A, Schiava Della N, Brizzi V, Arsicot M, Boudjelit T, Herail J, Feugier P, Lermusiaux P. The antegrade approach using transbrachial access improves technical success rate of endovascular recanalization of TASC C-D aortoiliac occlusion in case of failed femoral access. Ann Vasc Surg. 2015;29:1346–52.

13. Cortese B, Trani C, Lorenzoni R, Sbarzaglia P, Latib A, Tommasino A, Bovenzi F, Cremonesi A, Burzotta F, Pitì A, Tarantino F, Colombo A. Safety and feasibility of iliac endovascular interventions with a radial approach. Results from a multicenter study coordinated by the Italian Radial Force. Int J Cardiol. 2014;175:280–4.

14. Rogers RK, Tsai T, Casserly IP. Novel application of the "CART" technique for endovascular treatment of external iliac artery occlusions. Catheter Cardiovasc Interv. 2010;75:673–8.

15. Mwipatayi BP, Thomas S, Wong J, Temple SEL, Vijayan V, Jackson M, Burrows SA, Covered Versus Balloon Expandable Stent Trial (COBEST) Co-investigators. A comparison of covered

vs bare expandable stents for the treatment of aortoiliac occlusive disease. J Vasc Surg. 2011;54:1561–70.

16. Mendelsohn FO, Santos RM, Crowley JJ, Lederman RJ, Cobb FR, Phillips HR, Weissman NJ, Stack RS. Kissing stents in the aortic bifurcation. Am Heart J. 1998;136:600–5.

17. Scheinert D, Schröder M, Balzer JO, Steinkamp H, Biamino G. Stent-supported reconstruction of the aortoiliac bifurcation with the kissing balloon technique. Circulation. 1999;100:II295–300.

18. Yilmaz S, Sindel T, Golbasi I, Turkay C, Mete A, Lüleci E. Aortoiliac kissing stents: long-term results and analysis of risk factors affecting patency. J Endovasc Ther. 2006;13:291–301.

19. Mohamed F, Sarkar B, Timmons G, Mudawi A, Ashour H, Uberoi R. Outcome of "kissing stents" for aortoiliac atherosclerotic disease, including the effect on the non-diseased contra-lateral iliac limb. Cardiovasc Intervent Radiol. 2002;25:1–1.

20. Björses K, Ivancev K, Riva L, Manjer J, Uher P, Resch T. Kissingstents in the aortic bifurca-tion – a valid reconstruction for aorto-iliac occlusive disease. Eur J Vasc Endovasc Surg. 2008;36:424–31.

21. Haulon S, Mounier-Véhier C, Gaxotte V, Koussa M, Lions C, Haouari BA, Beregi JP. Percutaneous reconstruction of the aortoiliac bifurcation with the "kissing stents" tech-nique: long-term follow-up in 106 patients. J Endovasc Ther. 2002;9:363–8.

22. Sabri SS, Choudhri A, Orgera G, Arslan B, Turba UC, Harthun NL, Hagspiel KD, Matsumoto AH, Angle JF. Outcomes of covered kissing stent placement compared with bare metal stent placement in the treatment of atherosclerotic occlusive disease at the aortic bifurcation. JVIR. 2010;21:995–1003.

23. Krishnamurthy VN, Eliason JL, Henke PK, Rectenwald JE. Intravascular ultrasound-guided true lumen reentry device for recanalization of unilateral chronic total occlusion of iliac arter-ies: technique and follow-up. Ann Vasc Surg. 2010;24:487–97.

Chapter 3
Femoropopliteal Artery Chronic Total Occlusion Intervention

Subhash Banerjee and Emmanouil S. Brilakis

Femoropopliteal (FP) artery endovascular intervention procedures are one of the most common lower extremity peripheral artery interventions (PAI) worldwide. Chronic total occlusions are highly prevalent in this vascular bed and comprise nearly 40–50% of lesions treated [1]. Intervention on FP CTO lesions is technically more challenging, is an independent predictor of procedure failure, and is associated with higher complication rates compared with non-FP CTO procedures [2]. Therefore, a systematic and step-by-step approach to such lesions, along with familiarity with various PAI tools and their attributes, is crucial to successful PAI interventional practice. In this chapter we will review a step-by-step approach to FP CTO. Given the high likelihood of tackling such lesions in clinical practice, the ability to treat FP CTO is nearly obligatory for an endovascular specialist treating patients with peripheral artery disease (PAD).

The following topics are covered in this section:

1. Imaging FP CTO
2. Key definitions
3. Procedure planning
4. Vascular and lesion access
5. FP CTO crossing strategies
6. Treatment options for FP CTO lesions

Imaging FP CTO The diagnosis of FP CTO lesion in patients referred for clinically indicated endovascular treatment of PAD includes: duplex ultrasound (DUS), computed

S. Banerjee, MD (✉)
University of Texas Southwestern Medical Center and Veterans Affairs North Texas Health Care System, Dallas, TX, USA
e-mail: subhash.banerjee@utsouthwestern.edu

E.S. Brilakis
Minneapolis Heart institute, Minneapolis, MN, USA

University of Texas Southwestern Medical Center, Dallas, TX, USA
e-mail: esbrilakis@gmail.com

© Springer Science+Business Media Singapore 2017
S. Banerjee (ed.), *Practical Approach to Peripheral Arterial Chronic Total Occlusions*, DOI 10.1007/978-981-10-3053-6_3

tomography angiography (CTA), magnetic resonance angiography (MRA), and invasive contrast angiography (CA). CA is the most commonly used modality for diagnosis and procedure planning of FP CTO interventions. It allows optimal visualization of lower extremity (LE) peripheral artery anatomy, FP CTO lesion location, determination of lesion length, distal reconstitution (distal target), below-the-knee filling, vascularization of the feet, calcification, nature of the CTO stumps, collateral filling, and anatomy and tortuosity of contralateral iliac, profunda femoris, and pedal vessels. This information is crucial for planning a treatment strategy and vascular access. None of the other imaging modalities provide as complete and accurate information for planning FP CTO intervention as CA. However, the technique and quality of CA imaging is an important element and requires careful and deliberate attention. Imaging of inflow iliac and common femoral arteries is important, digital subtraction angiography (DAS) is preferred, and it is advisable to begin imaging sequence with an abdominal aortogram with the imaging frame set to capture at least 10–20 mm of the infrarenal aorta superior to the aortic bifurcation and both common femoral arteries. This would allow the operator to not only appreciate any aortoiliac disease and the steepness of the aortoiliac artery bifurcation, but also any accessory renal artery takeoffs from the common iliac arteries. Assessment of vascular calcification, tortuosity of the external iliacs, presence of prior iliac artery stents, and state of the profunda femoris origin provide tremendously important information for case planning. A marker pigtail catheter or a RIM catheter (AngioDynamics, Latham, NY) placed 10–20 mm above the aortoiliac bifurcation is optimal for this purpose, along with appropriate instructions to the patient and even a practice breath holding run to optimize DSA abdominal aortographic image capture (Fig. 3.1).

Following aortography, dropping the RIM catheter to engage the contralateral common iliac artery origin is the next best step. From here, there are two imaging options. One could inject into the common iliac artery and image the contralateral common femoral artery (CFA) bifurcation, panning down to capture mid and distal superficial femoral artery (SFA) angiograms, or rely on the image of the CFA bifurcation acquired during aortography and plan selective injection into of the CFA. The latter can be performed by advancing a supportive hydrophilic 0.035-inch guidewire (Glidewire

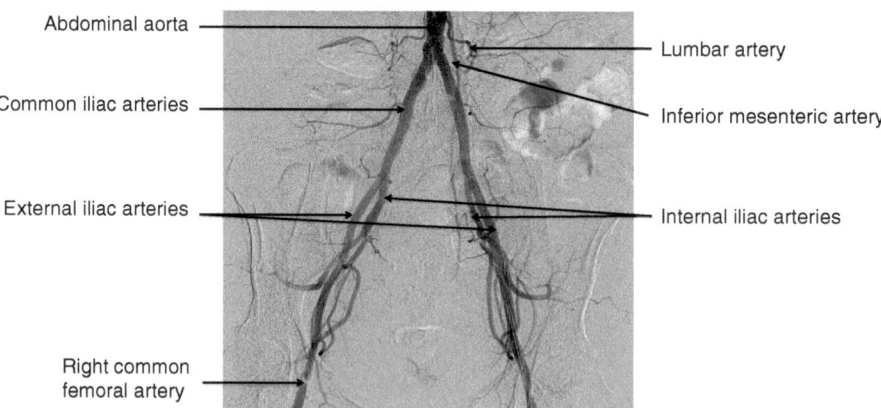

Fig. 3.1 Abdominal aortogram

Advantage; Somerset, NJ) through the RIM catheter into the distal SFA, or as far as possible, and advancing a straight tip end-hole 0.035-inch catheter (CXI; Bloomington, IN) into the SFA after withdrawing and exchanging out the RIM. Advancing the RIM catheter into the distal SFA is possible; however injecting contrast through its curved tip positioned against the vessel wall may result in SFA dissection and contrast staining. However, careful manipulation of the RIM and monitoring of arterial pressure tracing from its tip can be safely performed. Selective cannulation of the SFA allows FP and below-the-knee artery (BTK) angiography. Such angiography under DSA can often be performed with limited contrast (often 1:1–1:3 contrast to saline dilution) and provides high-quality angiograms of distal vessels. If abdominal aortography demonstrates occlusion of ostial or proximal SFA, selective angiography of the CFA with BTK and distal SFA imaging under DSA is the only alternative and helps determine distal FP reconstitution and/or BTK and distal foot perfusion. In patients with critical limb ischemia (CLI), delineation of pedal vessels is necessary. In claudicants, at least imaging up to the ankle vessels is highly recommended. It is best to set yourself up to image pedal vessels in all cases, and therefore selective DSA distal FP or BTK angiography is preferable to runoffs in the absence of proximal SFA occlusion.

CFA bifurcation anatomy is invariably symmetrical bilaterally, and often the origin of a SFA with flush ostial occlusion (no nub) can be estimated based on its contralateral takeoff or careful examination of the CFA bifurcation angiogram for linear calcification tracks that often follow an occluded SFA course. A medial origin of the profunda femoris to the SFA or a high bifurcation of CFA needs to be considered and can be infrequently encountered in clinical practice (Fig. 3.2). The inferior epigastric

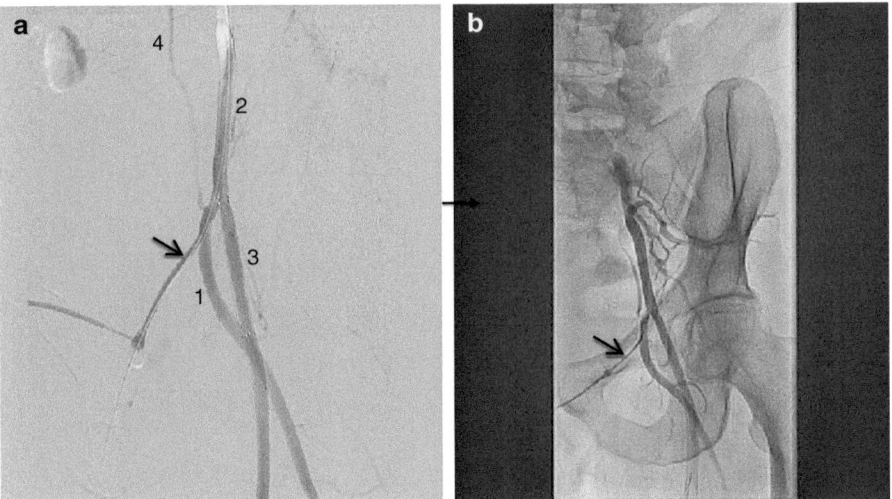

a and b: Illustrate medial origin of the profunda femoris artery (1) from the common femoral artery (2). The profunda femoris lies medial to the superficial femoral artery (3) and the inferior epigastric artery originated from the proximal profunda femoris artery (4).

Fig. 3.2 Anomalous origin of the profunda femoris artery. (**a, b**) Illustrate medial origin of the profunda femoris artery (*1*) from the common femoral artery (*2*). The profunda femoris lies medial to the superficial femoral artery (*3*) and the inferior epigastric artery originated from the proximal profunda femoris artery (*4*)

artery origin is an excellent guide to the intrapelvic boundary of the external iliac artery and is important to identify both at CFA access site angiography and contralateral CFA angiography. It is also an excellent landmark to know during antegrade access of the SFA. In the absence of optimal CFA vascular access during LE arterial angiography, brachial or radial artery angiography can often, from the left upper extremity, be accomplished with placement of pigtail catheter in the abdominal aorta as close as possible to the aortoiliac artery bifurcation. Anticoagulation during diagnostic angiography is not routinely needed; however unfractionated heparinization is recommended after placement of contralateral crossover sheath during a planned intervention. If a staged SFA intervention is being planned following an initial diagnostic catheterization performed earlier, at least repeating a series of diagnostic imaging of the SFA and BTK arteries is recommended to define the target lesion and BTK runoff. Moreover, such imaging is highly recommended if diagnostic images are suboptimal. Finally, attention needs to be directed to the profunda femoris artery, especially to its origin as profunda femoris PAD is often contiguous with ostial and proximal SFA and CFA atherosclerosis. It is vital to recognize that the profunda femoris artery supplies most collaterals to the LE and distal FP and BTK vessels, and avoiding injury, dissection or embolization, ostial plaque shift, or its obstruction with stents, devices, or sheaths is important and may result in acute ischemia of the LE and inadequate imaging of distal vessels. Early venous filling of the greater saphenous vein (most commonly) or other veins is also important to note as congenital and post-traumatic or postoperative SFA arteriovenous fistulous communications have been described, as have pseudoaneurysms of the SFA (Fig. 3.3).

Key Definitions Imaging of a SFA CTO begins with imaging of the proximal cap, delineation of collateral vessels and side branches, especially at the proximal and

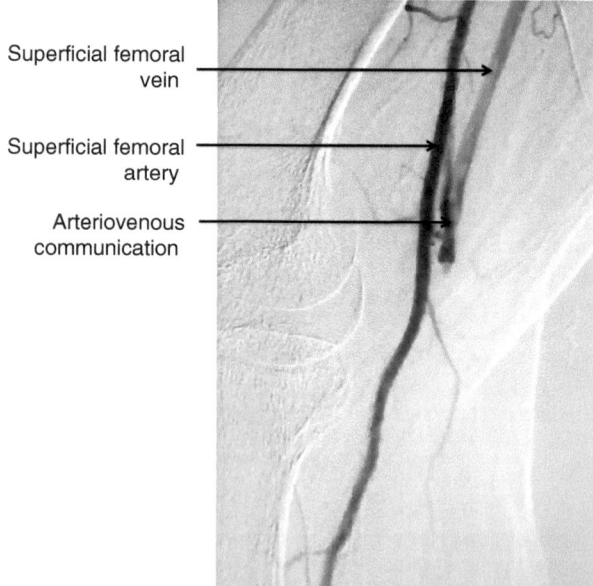

Superficial femoral vein

Superficial femoral artery

Arteriovenous communication

Fig. 3.3 Arteriovenous communication during SFA intervention. Illustrates an arteriovenous communication between the superficial femoral artery (SFA) and vein following successful recanalization of SFA chronic total occlusion

distal cap and the shape of the caps: blunt versus tapered. A CTO by definition has to be at least 3 months old, and, in the absence of prior imaging, a clinical definition is used that includes the presence of an occluded SFA without filling defects in the body of the occlusion to indicate more acute or subacute occlusion and no clinical history of acute onset of LE symptoms or other signs of acute limb ischemia (ALI) [3].

The key features of a FP CTO are indicated in Fig. 3.4. FP CTO length is defined by angiographic distance between the proximal and distal caps, and lesion length

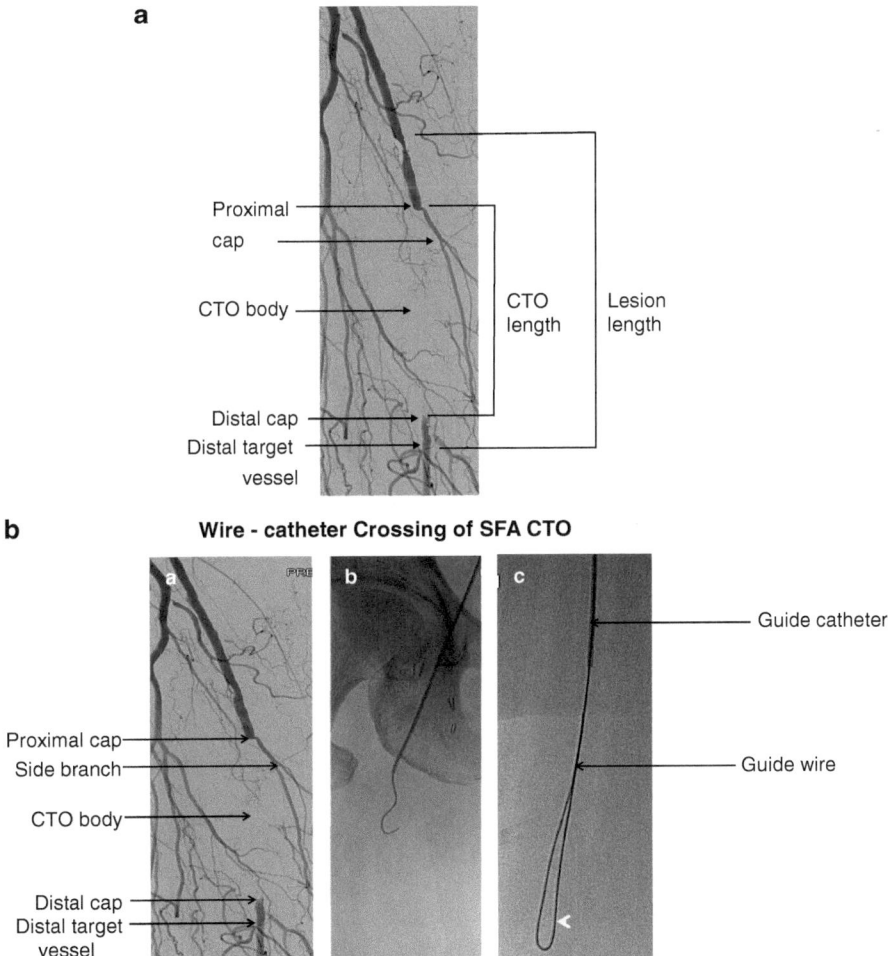

Fig. 3.4 (**a**) Features of femoropopliteal CTO. (**b**) Femoropopliteal CTO crossing. (*a*) Parts of a typical SFA CTO. (*b*) Inability to direct the wire in a SFA CTO. (*c*) Formation of a wire loop and passage advanced through the subintimal space. *Arrow head* indicates the width of the wire loop and the size of the potential subintimal space created

additionally includes any angiographic ≥70% diameter stenosis compared to the reference vessel segment. A single CTO is defined by angiographic 100% occlusion or sequential occlusions separated by ≤2 cm in the SFA and popliteal arteries or a single occlusion separated by ≤1 cm in BTK arteries. Vascular calcification visible on angiographic views prior to contrast injection is classified as mild (isolated foci of calcification), moderate (contiguous segments of calcification on one or alternating sides of the vessel), or severe (contiguous calcification on both sides of the vessel) [4].

Outcome measures include crossing success, procedure success, complications, and major adverse events (MAEs). Crossing success is defined as placement of a guidewire in the distal true lumen, past the distal CTO cap, confirmed by either angiography or intravascular ultrasound (IVUS) [4]. Crossing success can be primary (achieved with the initial CTO crossing strategy) (Fig. 3.5), secondary (failed initial strategy and subsequent success with an alternate device), or provisional (subintimal passage of the initial crossing device necessitating the use of a specialized reentry device). Procedure success is defined as successful revascularization of the CTO with ≤30% angiographic residual diameter stenosis [4]. Periprocedural complications included flow-limiting dissections, arterial perforations, access site hematomas ≥5 cm in diameter, retroperitoneal hematomas, distal embolization, major bleed requiring blood transfusion, or emergency surgery. MAE included all-cause mortality, nonfatal myocardial infarction, ischemic stroke, and unplanned endovascular or surgical revascularization/amputation of the target limb [5].

Procedure Plans Planning a FP CTO procedure requires recognition of patient, angiographic, and technical factors. Most FP CTO interventions are planned based on contrast angiographic images; however DUS, CTA, and/or MRA images can provide useful information that can often help the operator during case planning.

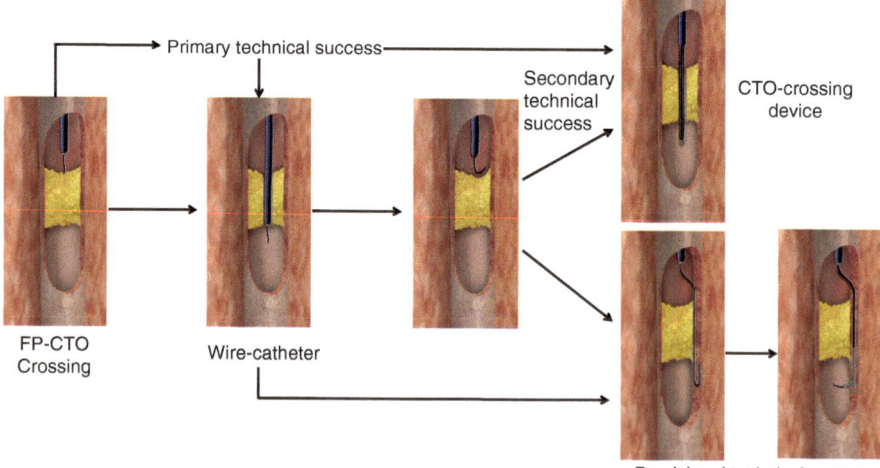

Fig. 3.5 Femoropopliteal CTO crossing strategies. Procedural success: successful revascularization of the CTO with a ≤30% residual diameter stenosis (My own figure from journal: needs copyright transfer *JEVT*)

Patient factors in FP CTO procedure planning include: symptom status, body habitus, renal function, chronic anticoagulation status, prior lower extremity vascular surgery or intervention, and compliance with medications, especially dual antiplatelet therapy (DAPT). Contralateral CFA access with retrograde sheath placement for SFA CTO intervention is the most common access with patient in supine position. Antegrade CFA access, although an attractive alternative as it reduces the distance to the FP CTO lesion, is technically more challenging especially in obese individuals, is associated with significantly higher vascular access complications, and requires repositioning and/or reorientation of the patient and equipment in the catheterization laboratory or vascular suite. It should be performed by experienced operators and after careful evaluation of the surface anatomy and preferably under ultrasound (US) guidance with micropuncture needle. For popliteal artery (PA) access, the patients should remain supine, with the lower extremity in a 60° external rotation and the knee in a gentle flexion. An angiogram via the proximal sheath should be performed to confirm the suitable level for distal PA puncture. In accordance with the standard surgical approach for the distal PA, the puncture site should be determined beforehand 8–10 cm below the border of the medial condyle of the femur and parallel with the posterior medial border of the tibia for 1 cm. Puncture should be performed with a 21-gauge micropuncture needle (Cook, Bloomington, Ind), obliquely from caudal to cranial. The C-arm should be adjusted for precise alignment with the axis of the puncture needle. Puncture is best performed under fluoroscopic guidance during live contrast. When access is obtained within the true lumen of the PA, a 0.018-inch V-18 guidewire (Boston Scientific, Natick, Mass) could be inserted, and the needle is pulled out.

For retrograde puncture of the distal right SFA, the C-arm has to be brought to a left anterior oblique position, and the needle has to form a line with the artery. To check the distance of the needle tip to the artery during puncturing, the C-arm should be brought into a right anterior oblique position at a 90° rotation from the previous one. Retrograde access should be obtained distal to the adductor canal. A V-18 Control guidewire could be passed through a 7-cm-long, 21-G needle.

Vascular and Lesion Access A 6 or 7F vascular access sheath inserted from contralateral common femoral access is most frequently employed for treating SFA CTO lesions. The sheath tip should be placed close to the SFA-popliteal artery bifurcation to provide maximum support for crossing catheters and guidewires. As one approaches a SFA CTO, there are numerous factors one could consider: presenting symptoms, lesion location, length, calcification, character of proximal and distal cap, collateral vessels, prior stent without fracture, multilevel occlusions, and distal vessel disease and flow. Figure 3.6 outlines four key steps that need to be defined prior to approaching a FP CTO lesion: lesion, approach, device, and strategy. Among all factors that should be considered, lesion length, features of the proximal cap, and level of distal reconstitution are most defining in outlining a crossing strategy and selection of crossing device [6]. Figure 3.7 depicts a simple classification of FP CTO lesions based on these key determinants and provides a guide to an

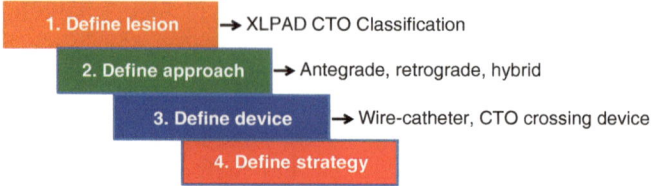

Fig. 3.6 XLPAD approach to femoropopliteal CTO: four key steps

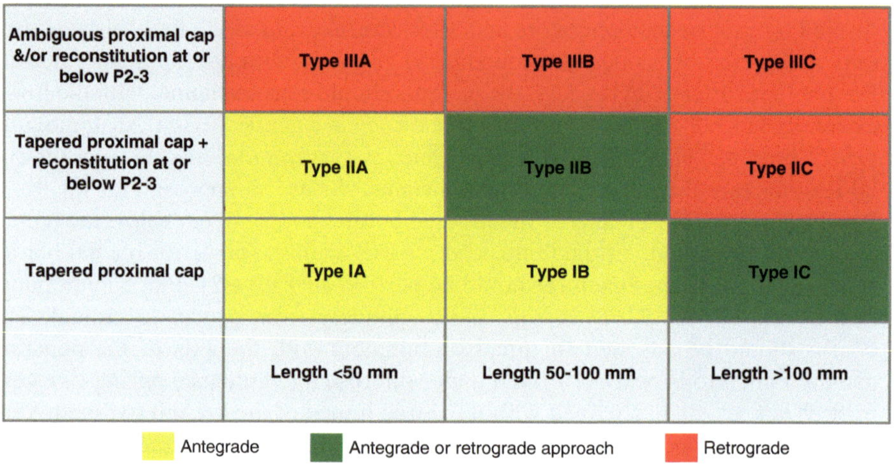

Ambiguous proximal cap &/or reconstitution at or below P2-3	Type IIIA	Type IIIB	Type IIIC
Tapered proximal cap + reconstitution at or below P2-3	Type IIA	Type IIB	Type IIC
Tapered proximal cap	Type IA	Type IB	Type IC
	Length <50 mm	Length 50-100 mm	Length >100 mm

⬜ Antegrade	🟩 Antegrade or retrograde approach	🟥 Retrograde

Fig. 3.7 Femoropopliteal CTO classification and initial crossing approach (Adapted from: Mustapha et al. [7])

initial crossing approach. Type I lesions have a tapered proximal cap that is most favorable for crossing device or guidewire engagement. Such lesions are classified as Type I lesions with Types IA, IB, and IC designating increasing CTO lesion lengths from <50 mm, 50–100 mm, and >100 mm, respectively. Type IA and IB can be approached antegrade with a guidewire-catheter or wire-catheter (WC) approach (Fig. 3.8). This systematic approach to tackle FP CTO lesions was first introduced by Mustapha et al. and was published as an abstract in 2014. We have modified it to include crossing device selection. For Type IC lesions, an antegrade or a retrograde approach should be considered, and a CTO crossing device (CCD) is preferred over WC in the presence of heavy fluoroscopic calcification. Detailed description of CTO crossing devices is provided in a dedicated chapter of this publication (Chap. 6). Careful attention to device, sheath and guidewire compatibility, should be paid prior to selection of a crossing strategy. Although comparative assessments of CCD and/or WC are absent, these recommendations are based on best-practice descriptions and consensus opinion. Type II lesions have a tapered proximal cap, however reconstitute at or below the P2–P3 arterial segments of the popliteal artery. Again, types IIA, IIB and IIC designate <50 mm, 50-100 mm, and >100 mm CTO lengths, respectively. Type IIA CTOs are likely to be accessed via an antegrade approach

Ambiguous proximal cap &/or reconstitution at or below P2-3	Type IIIA (WC); (CCD)*	Type IIIB (WC); (CCD)*	Type IIIC (WC); (CCD)*
Tapered proximal cap + reconstitution at or below P2-3	Type IIA (WC)	Type IIB (WC); (CCD)*	Type IIC (WC); (CCD)*
Tapered proximal cap	Type IA (WC)	Type IB (WC)	Type IC (WC); (CCD)*
	Length <50 mm	Length 50-100 mm	Length >100 mm

Antegrade Antegrade or retrograde approach Retrograde *Heavy calcification

WC: wire-catheter; CCD: CTO crossing device

Fig. 3.8 Femoropopliteal CTO classification and crossing device selection (Adapted from: Mustapha et al. [7])

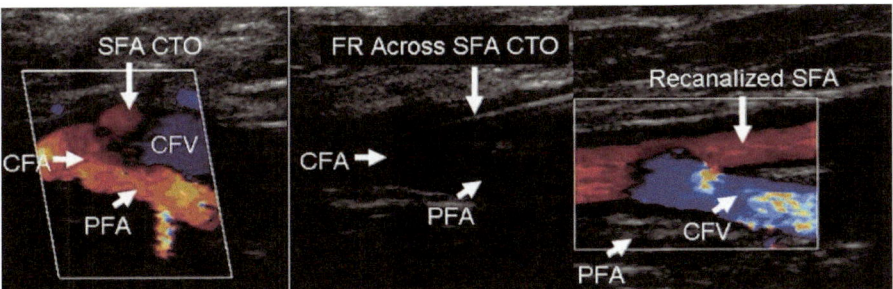

Fig. 3.9 Transcutaneous ultrasound-guided ostial SFA CTO crossing technique. *CFA* common femoral artery, *CFV* common femoral vein, *PFA* profunda femoral artery, *SFA* superficial femoral artery, *CTO* chronic total occlusion, *FR* frontrunner CTO crossing device (My own figure from journal: needs copyright transfer *CRM*)

predominantly with WC strategy; however Type IIB and IIC lesions could be crossed with WC or CCDs via antegrade or retrograde access points. Again, CCD should be preferred for heavily calcified lesions. FP CTO lesions with an ambiguous proximal cap and distal reconstitution involving below-the-knee vessels are particularly challenging and are classified as Type III FP CTO. Given the ambiguity of the proximal cap, a primary retrograde approach should be favored. For ostial SFA flush occlusions with no identifiable angiographic nub or proximal cap, a transcutaneous ultrasound-guided CTO puncture technique could also be used (Fig. 3.9).

Selection of guidewires and support catheters can be based on some basic principles. Polymer or plastic sleeves are applied on guidewires to enhance lubricity and reduce friction. These sleeves are designed to facilitate smooth tracking of the guidewires and improve lesion crossing. Guidewires also have applied coatings. Hydrophobic coatings are typically silicone based and repel water while enabling stronger tactile feedback. This tactile feedback is crucial during FP CTO crossing and required for navigating guidewires and maintaining an intraluminal course. Thus, hydrophobic guidewires have a lower tendency for subintimal passage. Guidewires with hydrophilic coatings that attract water and create a lubricious gel-like surface provide much lower friction and better trackability. These guidewires are best employed to navigate tortuous and severely stenosed vascular segments with minimal disruption of intraluminal thrombi. However, because these guidewires provide very limited tactile feedback, tend to loop, and easily dissect their way into the subintimal space, they are preferred during an intentional subintimal passage of the guidewire generally supported with a microcatheter. Tables 3.1 and 3.2 provide guidewire and support catheter options that are frequently employed in crossing FP CTO lesions.

FP CTO Crossing Strategies The intraluminal or IL FP CTO crossing technique is the most frequently employed, at least initially. A 0.014-, 0.018-, or 0.035-inch hydrophilic wire is frequently used in combination with a support catheter or a CCD. It is important to remember here that many CCDs require a 0.014- or 0.018-inch guidewire. A 0.035-inch guidewire and a compatible microcatheter with a straight or angled tip are most frequently used. The operator has to depend on tactile feedback provided by the WC combination and has to navigate based on the perceived course of the vessel based on fluoroscopic calcifications, collateral filling of a section of the vessel, and/or distal reconstitution. The catheter tip is maintained at close proximity to the wire tip, and care is taken not to allow the guidewire tip to

Table 3.1 Guidewire options for femoropopliteal CTO intervention

↓ Increasing tip penetration ↓		Boston Scientific	Cook	Cordis	Abbott	Terumo	Asahi
	0.014	Journey	Approach 6		Command		Miraclebros
		V-14	Approach 12		Pilot		Confianza
		Victory	Approach 18				Astato XS 20
			Approach 25				
	0.018	V-18			Connect		Astato 30
		Victory			Connect Flex		
		Treasure			Connect 250T		
	0.036					Glidewire	
						Advantage	

Grey: Standard hydrophilic guide wires
Green: Preferred CTO guide wires for FP CTO

Typical wire escalation strategy:
Treasure 12➔ Astato XS 20➔ Astato 30/Approach 25

Table 3.2 Support catheters for femoropopliteal CTO intervention

	Boston Scientific	Cook	Bard	Vascular solutions	Medtronic	Spectranetics	Terumo
0.014	Rubicon		Seeker	Minnie	Trailblazer	Quick-cross	
0.018	Rubicon	CXI	Seeker	Minnie	Trailblazer	Quick-cross	
0.035	Rubicon	CXI	Seeker	Minnie	Trailblazer	Quick-cross	Navicross

loop and dissect into the subintimal space [8]. Often, dilation of the proximal segments of the FP CTO may be required with a compatible undersized balloon to decrease friction and facilitate advancement of the support catheter over the guidewire. Intravascular ultrasound (IVUS) may be used to confirm intraluminal or subintimal location of the guidewire when the course is unreliable. In difficult to penetrate locations, a laser catheter may be used to ablate IL debris, and the guidewire is replaced either by a CCD with or without microcatheter support or by a hydrophilic looped wire technique used to traverse the lesion through a subintimal tract. Confirmation of distal vessel true lumen entry can be obtained with (a) free passage of the guidewire into the distal vessels, (b) contrast injection proximally or through the microcatheter following distal pressure recording, (c) easy aspiration of blood, (d) or by IVUS. IVUS should be preferred in difficult to cross lesions as it is most reliable and provides crucial information, not only about the location of the distal guidewire tip but also about the course of the guidewire along the body of the CTO. This information can be crucial in determining the subsequent treatment course, especially if debulking of the lesion with an atherectomy catheter is planned. Contrast injection through the microcatheter tip advanced across the distal CTO cap should be discouraged as it can be unreliable and, in rare situations, can propel distal hydraulic dissection and contrast staining of the interventional area making continuing with the procedure quite difficult.

The subintimal or SI technique is to proactively manipulate the WC to create a "neolumen" between the intimal and adventitial layers of the arterial wall. SI dissection technique is best employed with a 0.035-inch hydrophilic guidewire and compatible microcatheter [9]. The microcatheter is butted against the vessel wall or point of resistance, and the hydrophilic guidewire is advanced to create a loop. The catheter tip should be kept a short (10–20 mm) away from the guidewire, and both should be advanced in unison to maintain a narrow guidewire loop size that can be freely advanced along the SI space and perforate spontaneously back into the true lumen in the majority of cases at or beyond the distal reconstitution of the FP CTO. In about a third of cases, a specialized SI reentry device is needed to puncture a tract from the SI space into the true lumen of the distal vessel. The reentry device is generally delivered over the guidewire placed in the SI space, and it is recommended that a fresh guidewire be passed into the true lumen through the reentry device. Some devices, like the Enteer™, require a specialized preshaped wire with a probe for reentry (Stingray™). It is not uncommon that the subintimal tract is predilated with an undersized (generally 2.0 mm) balloon to facilitate delivery of more bulky reentry devices like the Outback™ or OffRoad™. Following successful distal vessel reentry, the reentry site needs to be optimally predilated as it may offer greater than expected resistance to delivery of larger sized balloons or stents.

IL CTO crossing is an easily acquired skill set and is the most commonly used CTO crossing method. It is an easy transition from crossing highly stenotic lesions and a well-understood translation for the interventionist. Furthermore, the procedural costs are quite low and limited to a standard guidewire and crossing catheter. Problems associated with the IL technique are that it is not uniformly successful and may require conversion to SI angioplasty to achieve a technically successful crossing. Without concurrent imaging, it is also difficult to know whether CTO crossing remains truly IL or the guidewire does not veer off segmentally into SI channels. Because of the amount of IL material, there is a frequent need to add adjunctive therapy other than a standard angioplasty balloon. This may require the addition of atherectomy devices or scoring balloons to debulk or modify the plaque. Stents may also be required to maintain an adequate flow channel. Unlike IL crossing, SI CTO crossing utilizes a WC approach that is significantly lower in cost compared to specialized CCDs. However, SI technique has a steeper learning curve and requires greater experience and training. In a third of SI cases, a specialized reentry device is required to reach the distal true lumen. Failure to reenter the true lumen is the most common cause of failure of this technique. Moreover, SI passage may also limit use of atherectomy catheters and is overall associated with higher complication rates, including perforation and loss of collateral vessels. Stenting is generally needed to secure SI crossing of FP CTOs.

3.1   Retrograde FP CTO Intervention

Crossing FP CTO via antegrade approach can be unsuccessful despite use of dedicated CCDs. Retrograde access could then be used to traverse the occluded segment. Retrograde access to the SFA can be obtained via the popliteal or pedal arteries [10]. Popliteal artery access requires the patient to be positioned in a prone position. It can be uncomfortable for the patient and inconvenient to implement during an ongoing procedure. Pedal access for retrograde FP intervention may provide marginal support and can be limited by the lengths of equipment available to treat the FP CTO. An alternative retrograde femoral artery approach that allows the patient to remain in a supine position has been described. For retrograde approach via the distal SFA, a 21-G at least 15-mm needle is recommended to penetrate the medial and ventral aspect of the patient's lower inner thigh corresponding to the SFA distal to the adductor canal. The puncture is performed under fluoroscopic guidance, and contrast injection through the sheath tip placed in the ipsilateral common femoral artery or proximal SFA may be needed. The C-arm should be first positioned in a contralateral oblique (30°–45°) position. For the right SFA, the C-arm should be in a left oblique position and vice versa. After making the puncture and advancing the needle through the thigh muscles, the C-arm should be moved to a 90° orthogonal position to confirm whether the needle is in line with the SFA when it is opacified with contrast. Once a coaxial position is confirmed, puncture of the distal SFA should be performed. After successful puncture, a 0.018-inch guidewire (V-18 Control; Boston Scientific, Natick, MA, USA) could be inserted through the needle followed by a 4 or 6F, 10-cm sheath (Terumo) or dedicated support catheter. Generally, a support catheter can be advanced retrograde through the occluded segment. In rare situations, a sheath needs to be inserted through the retrograde SFA puncture for delivery of CCDs. If advancement into the true lumen is not possible, a double-balloon inflation over antegrade and retrograde wires is advised to disrupt dissection planes and create a channel for antegrade or retrograde guidewire

Table 3.3 Factors for consideration during retrograde femoropopliteal CTO intervention

Clinical consideration	Anatomical consideration	Relative contraindications
Patients' presentation with critical limb ischemia	Adequate distal SFA, popliteal or tibial or pedal arteries	Last remaining below-the-knee vessel in claudicants
Long (≥100 mm) or multilevel femoropopliteal CTO	Patients with adequate anterior and posterior communicating circulation of the feet	Patients with contraindications to anticoagulation or arterial vasodilator drugs
Distal reconstitution of femoropopliteal CTO at or below the P2–P3 segment of the popliteal artery	Favorable distal CTO cap morphology	Absence of detectable adequate caliber below-the-knee arteries
Patients with hostile groin access (extensive scarring, morbid obesity, groin infection or wound), unable to lay flat		Inability to insert a sheath (may place retrograde guidewire to mark distal CTO target)

advancement into the true lumen of the SFA. Following access of the guidewire into the true lumen, externalization and preferably antegrade delivery of balloons and stents is necessary to complete the CTO recanalization procedure. A comparison of antegrade and retrograde FP intervention is depicted in Table 3.3. Generally, the retrograde access catheter can be removed and pressure applied externally to achieve hemostasis. Occasionally, balloon occlusion of the SFA puncture site over a guidewire placed within the vessel is needed. A case of anterior tibial artery and retrograde SFA stent puncture is depicted in Fig. 3.10a, b.

3.2 Transcutaneous Ultrasound-Guided Endovascular Crossing of FP CTO

3.2.1 Peripheral Arterial Segments

Crossing of long and complex infra-inguinal arterial CTO presents a significant challenge, and inability to remain intraluminal or reenter the true lumen after subintimal dissection is the main reason for procedural failures and complications. A novel technique has been described for endovascular crossing of complex infra-inguinal CTOs using frontrunner blunt microdissection (FR) with transcutaneous ultrasound guidance (TUG) [11]. The technique was used to cross two long SFA CTOs (left, 300 mm; right, 140 mm) in patients with chronic kidney disease. TUG allowed: (a) accurate visualization of occluded SFA segments (Fig. 3.9) and the echo-reflective FR catheter, (b) directional control and safe intraluminal manipulation of FR avoiding subintimal entry, (c) confirmation of distal true lumen access, and (d) hemodynamic assessment after stenting. The above were

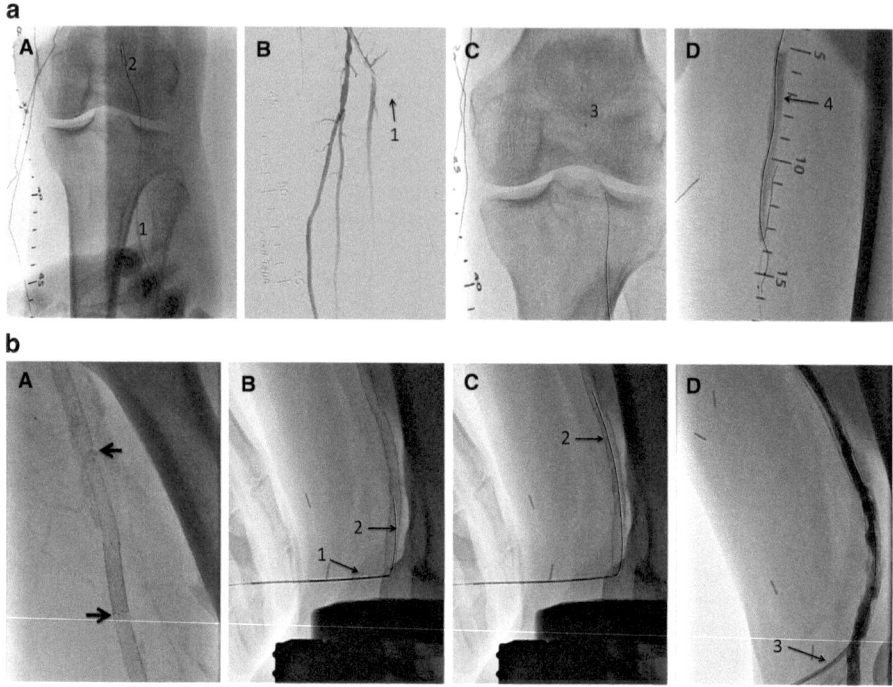

Fig. 3.10 (**a**) Retrograde anterior tibial artery CTO intervention of the SFA. (*A*) Illustrates anterior tibial artery access and insertion of 6F sheath (*1*) over 0.018-inch guidewire (*2*); (*B*) sheath in anterior tibial artery; (*C*) a leading 0.014-inch crossing catheter (*3*) advanced in retrograde fashion through the distal popliteal artery CTO cap supported with an appropriate guidewire; (*D*) dilation of the subintimal tract with balloon (*4*) to facilitate retrograde entry of the guidewire into true lumen. (**b**) Retrograde SFA stent puncture. (*A*) Illustrates stent fractures in the superficial femoral artery or SFA (*bold arrows*); (*B*) medial thigh puncture with microneedle (*1*) and 0.018-inch guidewire (*2*) advanced into the distal SFA (*C*); SFA angiogram via 6F sheath inserted in the distal SFA via retrograde medial thigh puncture of the SFA (*D*); Distal SFA angiogram with contrast injection through retrograde sheath (*3*)

achieved with minimal use of fluoroscopy and radiocontrast administration. This novel, simple, and reproducible technique can improve both the success and safety of endovascular intraluminal crossing of infra-inguinal arterial CTOs: TUG-CTO technique.

3.2.2 Transcollateral Approach to Femoropopliteal CTO

Presence of a large collateral at the proximal cap often makes penetration of the cap challenging. The crossing device or guidewire tends to slip into the collateral vessel and can also cause its dissection or perforation. Moreover, SI approach in the presence of a large collateral vessel at the SFA CTO proximal cap includes the risk of losing flow in the collateral. This is especially critical in the setting of an ostial SFA CTO with profunda femoral artery supply to the distal limb. A transcollateral approach to penetrate the distal CTO cap and either to cross retrograde, provide a distal target, or create a dissection plane with transcollateral small balloon delivery and distal cap angioplasty can facilitate crossing success [12]. A 0.014-inch 300-cm guidewire Asahi Fielder wire (Abbott) and a 0.14″ Quick-Cross catheter are generally best for traversing the collateral vessel. Selective injection can then be performed of the collateral vessel through the Quick-Cross. The Fielder wire is then advanced to the distal CTO cap the 0.14″ Quick-Cross moved to the distal SFA CTO cap over the guidewire. At this point, the Fielder wire can be switched to a Confianza Pro 12 guidewire (Abbott) to penetrate the distal cap. The Treasure 12 wire (Boston Scientific) can also be used to penetrate the cap. If attempts to advance the guidewire via the retrograde transcollateral approach are not possible, a small balloon (2.0 × 100 Coyote balloon, Boston Scientific) could be advanced via the collateral into the lesion in a retrograde manner. Following predilation via a retrograde approach, a soft guidewire can then be advanced distally from the antegrade approach.

3.2.3 "SAFARI" Technique

The "SAFARI" or subintimal arterial flossing with antegrade-retrograde intervention is a technique for recanalization of FP CTOs that can be employed when subintimal angioplasty is unsuccessful and retrograde access is feasible [13]. Retrograde access is usually obtained via the popliteal, distal anterior tibial artery, dorsalis pedis, or distal posterior tibial arteries.

3.2.4 Hybrid Approach to Femoropopliteal CTO Intervention

An optimal approach to FP CTO intervention involves thorough evaluation of baseline angiogram and the technical ability and expertise to switch from one technique to another. The hybrid approach to FP CTO intervention outlines some basic principles that need to be considered and employed to achieve reproducible success in crossing FP CTOs. The hybrid approach described here is based on an expert consensus and needs to be validated by ongoing research in this area. The goal of developing the hybrid approach is to demystify the procedure and make its underlying principle reproducible so that the broader interventional community can adopt it. It is also important to recognize that most CTO procedures of the SFA should be planned in advance and ad hoc intervention of FP CTOs should be strongly discouraged. As has been outlined earlier in this chapter, the first step of a hybrid approach to femoral popliteal CTO intervention is to clearly identify all sections of the

vascular anatomy. This can be achieved by delayed imaging of the distal reconstitution of the SFA or popliteal arteries or by dual injections simultaneously from proximal and distal vessels or via collateral vessels. An antegrade approach with guidewire
escalation along with a support catheter is the first step when the proximal cap is
tapered and favorable for penetration. The presence of a blunt cap, large collateral
vessel, heavy calcification, and/or fractured stent would require consideration of a
retrograde approach. Figure 3.11 depicts the hybrid approach to FP CTO. For long
FP CTO, the antegrade WC approach may render the guidewire in the SI space.
There are a few techniques that the operator should be aware of when accessing the
distal true lumen. Similarly, there are retrograde dissection-reentry techniques.
These techniques are outlined in Fig. 3.12. As part of an antegrade approach, the
looped guidewire could be advanced through the dissection plane till it enters the
distal true lumen as part of the subintimal tracking and reentry technique or STAR
technique. Although this technique is easy to execute, especially if the guidewire

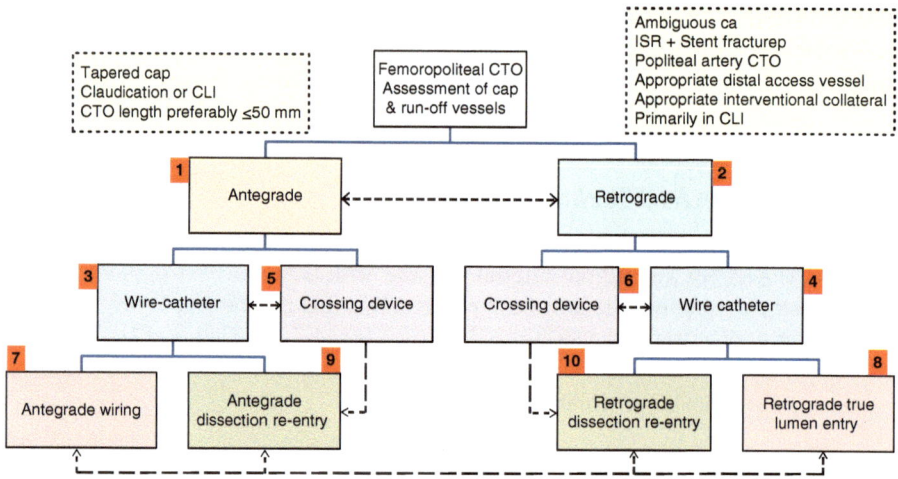

Fig. 3.11 Hybrid algorithm for crossing femoropopliteal CTO

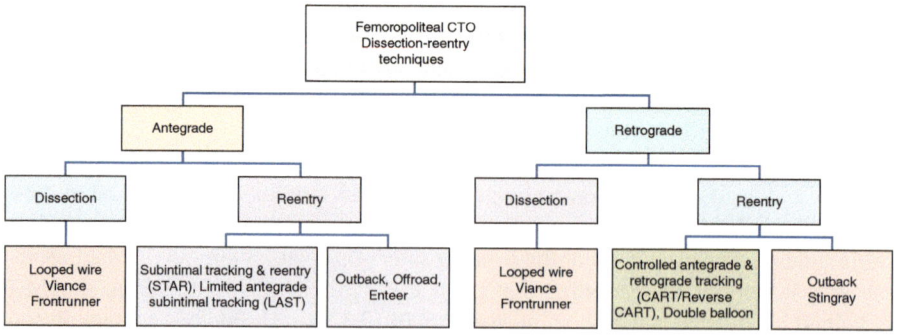

Fig. 3.12 Dissection-reentry techniques for crossing femoropopliteal CTO

loop is kept narrow, it can and often will close off collateral vessels that may make visualization of the distal reconstituted vessels poor as the case progresses if any of the lost collaterals significantly contributed to distal vessel filling. A limited antegrade subintimal or LAST technique often relies on a more limited antegrade dissection and is therefore less likely to cause significant loss of collaterals. If the above techniques fail, a dedicated reentry device should be used to reenter the distal true lumen. The selection of the type of reentry device is often guided by the guidewire support, angulation of the iliac bifurcation, sheath size, diameter of the subintimal space, ability to track or predilate the subintimal space, and, finally, expertise and familiarity of the operator. Use of dedicated reentry devices also contributes significantly to procedure cost. Often, an IVUS catheter may be used to determine the course of the guidewire and the point of its deviation into the subintimal space. A more supportive reentry device like the Outback can also assist with a stepwise approach from the dissection plane toward the distal true lumen by performing multiple successive reentries. From a retrograde approach, as described earlier in the transcollateral technique, a balloon can be inflated in a retrograde dissection plane communicating with the distal true lumen to facilitate antegrade passage of the guidewire into the true lumen. This technique is called controlled antegrade-retrograde dissection/reentry or CART [14]. The CART technique can be applied to dilate the antegrade dissection space and is referred to as the reverse CART technique. A double-balloon technique can also be used to dilate via both antegrade and retrograde wires. However, care must be taken to not overlap the balloon tips that should be kept at about 5 mm from each other. Operators, as part of the hybrid approach, should be able to seamlessly switch from one technique to another. A comparative assessment of antegrade or retrograde approach to FP CTO is presented in Table 3.1. Tables 3.2 and 3.3 outline workhorse and preferred FP CTO guidewires and support catheters, along with a recommended guidewire escalation strategy.

References

1. Banerjee S, Pershwitz G, Sarode K, Mohammad A, Abu-Fadel MS, Baig MS, Tsai S, Little BB, Gigliotti OS, Soto-Cora E, Foteh MI, Rodriguez G, Klein A, Addo T, Luna M, Shammas NW, Prasad A, Brilakis ES. Stent and non-stent based outcomes of infrainguinal peripheral artery interventions from the multicenter XLPAD registry. J Invasive Cardiol. 2015;27(1):14–8.
2. Yang X, Lu X, Li W, Huang Y, Huang X, Lu M, Jiang M. Endovascular treatment for symptomatic stent failures in long-segment chronic total occlusion of femoropopliteal arteries. J Vasc Surg. 2014;60(2):362–8.
3. Banerjee S, Hadidi O, Mohammad A, Alsamarah A, Thomas R, Sarode K, Garg P, Baig MS, Brilakis ES. Blunt microdissection for endovascular treatment of infrainguinal chronic total occlusions. J Endovasc Ther. 2014;21(1):71–8.
4. Banerjee S, Sarode K, Patel A, Mohammad A, Parikh R, Armstrong EJ, Tsai S, Shammas NW, Brilakis ES. Comparative assessment of guidewire and microcatheter vs a crossing device-based strategy to traverse infrainguinal peripheral artery chronic total occlusions. J Endovasc Ther. 2015;22(4):525–34.

5. Banerjee S, Sarode K, Mohammad A, Gigliotti O, Baig MS, Tsai S, Shammas NW, Prasad A, Abu-Fadel M, Klein A, Armstrong EJ, Jeon-Slaughter H, Brilakis ES, Bhatt DL. Femoropopliteal artery stent thrombosis: report from the excellence in peripheral artery disease registry. Circ Cardiovasc Interv. 2016;9(2):e002730.
6. Clark TW, Groffsky JL, Soulen MC. Predictors of long-term patency after femoropopliteal angioplasty: results from the STAR registry. J Vasc Interv Radiol. 2001;12(8):923–33.
7. Mustapha JA, Saab F, Diaz-Sandoval L, McGoff T, Heaney C, Saad H. Chronic total occlusion crossing based on cap morphology (C-TOP) in CLI patients: a pilot study and interim analysis of the PRIME registry. Vascular Disease Management, September 2014, p. 219.
8. Yilmaz S, Sindel T, Yegin A, Lüleci E. Subintimal angioplasty of long superficial femoral artery occlusions. J Vasc Interv Radiol. 2003;14(8):997–1010.
9. Fanelli F, Cannavale A. Retrograde recanalization of complex SFA lesions indications and techniques. J Cardiovasc Surg 2014;55(4):465–71. Epub 2014 Jun 11.
10. Schmidt A, Bausback Y, Piorkowski M, Werner M, Bräunlich S, Ulrich M, Varcoe R, Friedenberger J, Schuster J, Botsios S, Scheinert D. Retrograde recanalization technique for use after failed antegrade angioplasty in chronic femoral artery occlusions. J Endovasc Ther. 2012;19(1):23–9.
11. Banerjee S, Das TS, Brilakis ES. Transcutaneous ultrasound-guided endovascular crossing of infrainguinal chronic total occlusions. Cardiovasc Revasc Med. 2010;11(2):116–9.
12. Werner GS, Coenen A, Tischer KH. Periprocedural ischaemia during recanalisation of chronic total coronary occlusions: the influence of the transcollateral retrograde approach. EuroIntervention. 2014;10(7):799–805.
13. Hua WR, Yi MQ, Min TL, Feng SN, Xuan LZ, Xing J. Popliteal versus tibial retrograde access for subintimal arterial flossing with antegrade-retrograde intervention (SAFARI) technique. Eur J Vasc Endovasc Surg. 2013;46(2):249–54.
14. Shi W, Yao Y, Wang W, Yu B, Wang S, Que H, Xiang H, Li Q, Zhao Q, Zhang Z, Xu J, Liu X, Shen L, Xing J, Wang Y, Shan W, Zhou J. Combined antegrade femoral artery and retrograde popliteal artery recanalization for chronic occlusions of the superficial femoral artery. J Vasc Interv Radiol. 2014;25(9):1363–8.

Chapter 4
Treatment of Femoropopliteal CTO

Subhash Banerjee

The Trans-Atlantic Inter-Society Consensus (TASC) II class D femoral/popliteal lesions include chronic total occlusions (CTOs) of the superficial femoral artery (SFA) that are >20 cm in length or involve the popliteal artery. Primary stenting has proven superior to percutaneous transluminal balloon angioplasty (PTA) for FP CTOs [1]. Table 4.1 provides an overview of currently recommended treatment strategies of FP peripheral artery disease. Although surgical treatment may be preferred, current advancement of endovascular techniques and devices has made peripheral vascular intervention (PVI) often the first-line approach. Overall there are limited dedicated studies on stent versus non-stent approaches to FP CTOs. Treatment strategies for long occlusions of the SFA following successful recanalization have not been standardized, although these occlusions are frequently encountered in clinical practice. Stenting often leads to exaggerated neointimal hyperplasia leading to high in-stent restenosis rates (10–40% at 6–24 months) and stent fractures [2]. The subintimal approach can contribute to insufficient dilation and recoil after stent placement in the subintimal space, whereas the response to balloon dilation and self-expandable stenting can be more predictable and favorable with an intraluminal approach.

Subintimal angioplasty is widely used for crossing of long CTO of the SFA with favorable immediate and late outcomes. Despite the frequent use of subintimal angioplasty for CTO lesions of the SFA, the role of stenting in the subintimal tract is unclear. Hong et al. recently reported outcomes of spot stenting versus long stenting after intentional subintimal approach for long chronic total occlusions of the femoropopliteal artery [3]. A total of 196 limbs in 163 patients, implanted with bare nitinol stents after subintimal approach in long femoropopliteal occlusions (lesion length 25 ± 8 cm), were retrospectively analyzed. The primary patency was com-

S. Banerjee, MD
University of Texas Southwestern Medical Center and Veterans Affairs North Texas Health Care System, Dallas, TX, USA
e-mail: subhash.banerjee@utsouthwestern.edu

© Springer Science+Business Media Singapore 2017
S. Banerjee (ed.), *Practical Approach to Peripheral Arterial Chronic Total Occlusions*, DOI 10.1007/978-981-10-3053-6_4

Table 4.1 Treatment indications for lower extremity PAD lesions

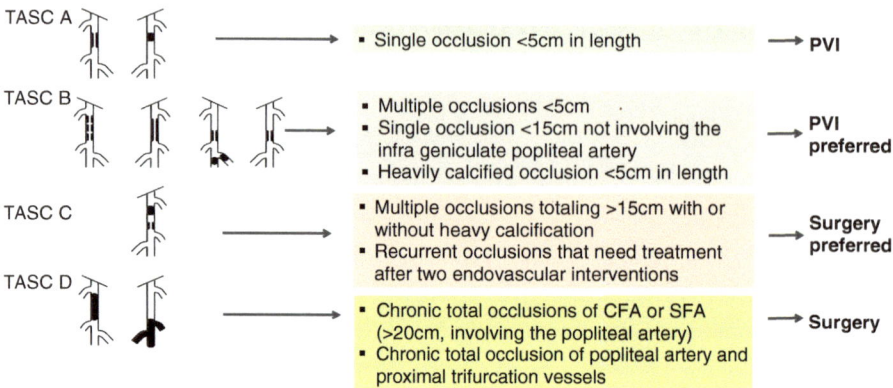

PVI peripheral vascular intervention
Norgren et al. [9]

pared between spot stenting ($n = 129$) and long stenting ($n = 67$). Adjusted-primary patency (47% vs. 77%, $p < 0.001$) and adjusted freedom from target lesion revascularization (52% vs. 84%, $p < 0.001$) at 2 years were significantly lower in the long stenting group than in the spot stenting group.

A complete intraluminal SFA CTO revascularization strategy may improve patency rates and clinical outcomes relative to subintimal technique. Matsumi et al. evaluated complete intraluminal angioplasty and self-expandable nitinol stenting for TASC II D SFA CTOs in 72 consecutive limbs of 68 patients [6]. Mean CTO length was 24.4 cm and ~50% of patients had a single-vessel below-the-knee runoff. Primary patency was 78% at 1 year, 70% at 2–3 years, and 52% at 5 years. These patency rates compare favorably to previously published patency rates in complex TASC II D SFA lesions, reported to 60% at 1 year, 20–50% at 2 years, and <50% at 3 years.

Kruse et al. reported 5-year outcome of patients treated with self-expanding covered stents for SFA occlusive disease and identify parameters that could predict loss of primary patency [7]. In this dual-center study, 315 consecutive patients (mean age 69.0±10.1 years; 232 men) were treated for SFA occlusive disease in 334 limbs with VIABAHN self-expanding covered stents between 2001 and 2014 and retrospectively analyzed. Mean lesion length was 11.7±8.8 cm. All-cause mortality at 5 years was 14.1%. Primary patency rates at 1, 3, and 5 years were 72.2%, 51.8%, and 47.6%, respectively, with secondary patency rates of 86.2%, 78.7%, and 77.5%. Covered stent diameter <7 cm was an independent predictor of loss of primary patency.

The evidence of use of drug-coated stent in patients with TASC C/D de novo femoropopliteal lesions is not conclusively in favor of stenting. In a recent single-center registry, patients were prospectively followed by clinical and ultrasound evaluation following FP CTO treatment with paclitaxel-coated stents. X-ray of the stented zone was systematically performed 12 months after implantation [6]. The primary endpoint was primary sustained clinical improvement after 12 months. One year primary sustained clinical improvement rates for claudication/CLI patients were $68.0\% \pm 9.3\%$ and $41.6\% \pm 11.1\%$, respectively ($p = 0.13$). The incidence of in-stent restenosis and stent thrombosis was 25% and 14%, respectively. The incidence of stent fracture was 12.5% per limb and 9% per implanted stent.

In the 1-year results of paclitaxel-coated balloons for long femoropopliteal artery disease (SFA-long study), the mean treated lesion length was 251 ± 71 mm, including 63.4% moderate to severely calcified lesions and 49.5% total occlusions [7]. The bailout stent rate was 10.9%. Follow-up after 12 months was obtained in 101 patients (96.2%), showing that primary patency was maintained in 84 (83.2%), and major adverse events had occurred in 7 (6.2%), with persistently significant clinical benefits in Rutherford class.

Also, drug-coated balloons combined with spot stenting may be advantageous for the treatment of long femoropopliteal CTO recanalization [8]. The placement of a new self-expanding interwoven nitinol stent (SUPERA, IDEV Technologies, Webster, Texas) or VIABAHN (Bard) may be another favorable option for the treatment of popliteal lesions. Overall, a wide spectrum of endovascular treatment options exists; the following successful FP CTO crossing (preferably intraluminal) is achieved. These include PTA with conventional balloons, drug-coated balloons, or "specialty" balloons (e.g., cutting, AngioSculpt scoring, or Chocolate balloons), primary or bailout nitinol or drug-eluting stent implantation, interwoven nitinol or PTFE-covered stents, and plaque modification by means of atherectomy. Despite these options, high-quality randomized clinical trial, comparative effectiveness, and cost-effectiveness data for treating FP CTOs are lacking, and specific studies in this area are urgently needed.

4.1 Follow-up of Patients Following Successful Femoropopliteal CTO

4.1.1 Intervention

Although no formally tested recommendations are lacking, our own practice is that patients should be observed at 1 month after the procedure and then examined at 6-month intervals up to a year. Noninvasive hemodynamic evaluations are repeated at 6 months and 1 year or if the symptom status deteriorates. At least one imaging study, such as CT angiography, duplex ultrasound, or intra-arterial angiography, is performed in the event of either a >0.15 decrement in the ABI or worsening symptoms that were reflected by changes in the Rutherford category.

References

1. Goetz JP, Kleemann M. Complex recanalization techniques for complex femoro-popliteal lesions: how to optimize outcomes. J Cardiovasc Surg. 2015;56:31–41.
2. Kasapis C, Henke PK, Chetcuti SJ, et al. Routine stent implantation vs percutaneous transluminal angioplasty in femoropopliteal artery disease: a meta analysis of randomized controlled trials. Eur Heart J. 2009;30:44–55.
3. Hong SJ, Ko YG, Shin DH, Kim JS, Kim BK, Choi D, Hong MK, Jang Y. Outcomes of spot stenting versus long stenting after intentional subintimal approach for long chronic total occlusions of the femoropopliteal artery. JACC Cardiovasc Interv. 2015;8(3):472–80.
4. Micari A, Vadalà G, Castriota F, Liso A, Grattoni C, Russo P, Marchese A, Pantaleo P, Roscitano G, Cesana BM, Cremonesi A. 1-year results of paclitaxel-coated balloons for long femoropopliteal artery disease: evidence from the SFA-long study. JACC Cardiovasc Interv. 2016;9(9):950–6.
5. Davaine JM, Querat J, Kaladji A, Guyomarch B, Chaillou P, Costargent A, Quillard T, Gouëffic Y. Treatment of TASC C and D Femoropoliteal Lesions with Paclitaxel eluting Stents: 12 month Results of the STELLA-PTX Registry. Eur J Vasc Endovasc Surg. 2015;50(5):631–7.
6. Matsumi J, Ochiai T, Tobita K, et al. Long-term outcomes of self-expandable nitinol stent implantation with intraluminal angioplasty to treat chronic total occlusion in the superficial femoral artery (TransAtlantic Inter-Society Consensus Type D lesions). J Invasive Cardiol. 2016;28:58–64.
7. Kruse RR, Poelmann FB, Doomernik D, Burgerhof HG, Fritschy WM, Moll FL, Reijnen MM. Five-year outcome of self-expanding covered stents for superficial femoral artery occlusive disease and an analysis of factors predicting failure. J Endovasc Ther 2015;22(6):855–61.
8. Zeller T, Rastan A, Macharzina R, et al. Drugcoated balloons vs. drug-eluting stents for treatment of long femoropopliteal lesions. J Endovasc Ther. 2014;21:359–68.
9. Norgren L et al. Inter-Society Consensus for the Management of Peripheral Arterial Disease (TASC II). J Vasc Surg. 2007;45(Suppl S):S5–67.

Chapter 5
Endovascular Treatment of Below-the-Knee Chronic Total Occlusions

Anand Prasad and Fadi Saab

5.1 Introduction

With the aging of the US population as well as the epidemic of obesity, metabolic syndrome, and diabetes, it is expected that lower extremity peripheral arterial disease (PAD) and specifically critical limb ischemia (CLI) will continue to be a major healthcare challenge. Although a full discussion of the epidemiology and pathophysiology of CLI is beyond the scope of this chapter, a few points will help provide perspective for the reader. An important concept to convey is that the relationship between diabetes and CLI is not *casual*, but rather *causal* in nature. The associations between diabetic prevalence, complications, and mortality track closely with the rates of CLI and of nontraumatic amputations. Over the course of a lifetime, a diabetic patient is significantly more likely to undergo limb loss than a nondiabetic – with over 60% of nontraumatic amputations being performed in diabetic individuals. Although the pathophysiology leading to CLI in these patients is multifactorial – neuropathy, deformity, impaired immune response, and inflammation – the role of diffuse below-the-knee (BTK) atherosclerosis remains central to the failure of healing of foot ulcers. Traditionally, diabetic foot ulcers were classified as neuropathic or ischemic in nature. We now know that 50% of "neuropathic" ulcers may have impaired healing due to underlying ischemia. This ischemia is often microvascular, but in many cases due to distal BTK disease involving the plantar circulation.

A term proposed to replace the traditional dichotomy of foot ulcer classification and provide better emphasis on the pathophysiology is the "neuro-ischemic ulcer" (Fig. 5.1) [1].

Given that progression of CLI to limb loss is multifactorial, a multidisciplinary approach is key to successful outcomes. A team of individuals addressing diabetes, infection, deformity, and wound bed care including hyperbaric therapy are needed.

A. Prasad, MD (✉) • F. Saab, MD
University of Texas Health Science Center, Department of Medicine,
Division of Cardiology, San Antonio, TX, USA
e-mail: anandprasadmd@gmail.com

© Springer Science+Business Media Singapore 2017
S. Banerjee (ed.), *Practical Approach to Peripheral Arterial Chronic Total Occlusions*, DOI 10.1007/978-981-10-3053-6_5

45

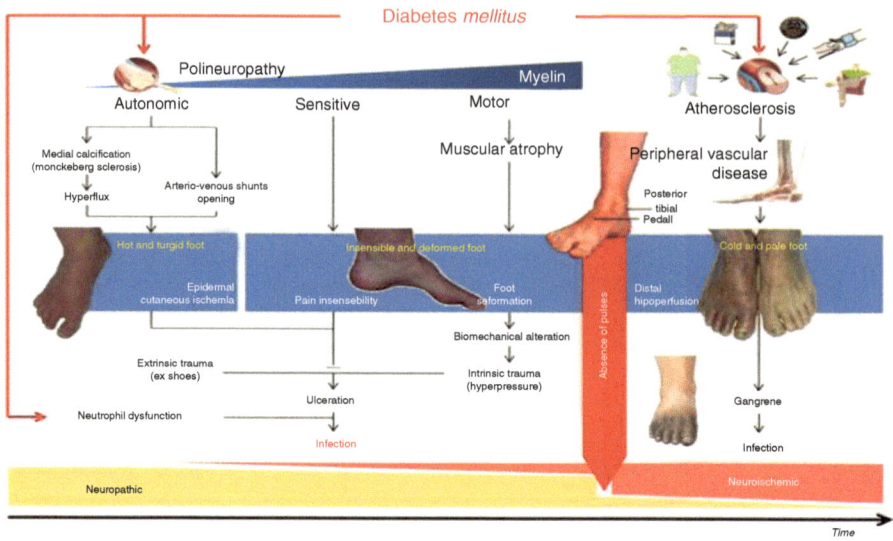

Fig. 5.1 Concept of the neuro-ischemic ulcer (From: Mendes and Neves [1])

However, a central tenant in CLI therapy is that despite supportive therapies a wound is unlikely to heal without restoration of arterial circulation – and conversely revascularization alone without adequate wound care and risk factor modification may also lead to suboptimal outcomes. The evaluation for the presence of ischemia is therefore paramount in any foot ulcer which is new, recurrent, fails to heal, or stalls in its healing process. The objective assessment of ischemia in the context of CLI remains challenging and controversial – and certainly again beyond the scope of this discussion. Often multiple modalities including transcutaneous oximetry, skin perfusion pressures, noninvasive anatomic imaging, and most importantly clinical judgment of patient risk factors and history must be employed [2]. It is this authors' belief that in the appropriate clinical scenario a low threshold must be in place for using selective catheter-based angiography to evaluate the lower extremity circulation – particularly the plantar vessels in patients with nonhealing foot ulcers [3]. Published data would suggest that revascularization results in higher rates of limb salvage, reduced ulcer recurrence, and perhaps reduced mortality as compared to "conservative therapy" [4, 5]. The decline in major amputations in the United States over the past decade has been linked to the rise in revascularization for CLI – particularly endovascular-based therapies. Despite these data, the vast majority of Americans with PAD still undergo a major amputation without angiography or attempt at revascularization [6].

5.2   BTK CTOs: Indications and Treatment Options

The presence of CLI remains the primary indication for revascularization of below-the-knee (BTK) vessels – including recanalization of chronic total occlusions (CTO). More controversial but potentially appropriate in specific situations is the

Table 5.1 Consensus statement of the Society of Cardiovascular Angiography and Interventions for clinical scenarios in which treatment of infrapopliteal (IP) artery disease may be considered

Recommendation	Clinical scenario
Appropriate care	Moderate–severe claudication (RC 2–3) with two- or three-vessel IP disease (if the arterial target lesion is focal)
	Ischemic rest pain (RC 4) with two- or three-vessel IP disease (to provide direct flow to the plantar arch and to maximize volume flow to foot)
	Minor tissue loss (RC 5) with two- or three-vessel IP disease (to provide direct flow to the plantar arch and to maximize volume flow to foot)
	Major tissue loss (RC 6) with two- or three-vessel IP disease (to prevent major amputation and to facilitate healing a minor amputation)
May be appropriate care	Moderate–severe claudication (RC 2–3) with two- or three-vessel IP disease (occlusion or diffuse disease)
	Ischemic rest pain (RC 4) with one- or two-vessel IP disease (to provide direct flow to the plantar arch and in two-vessel, to maximize volume flow to foot)
	Minor tissue loss (RC 5) with one-vessel IP disease (to provide direct flow to the plantar arch and to maximize volume flow to foot)
Rarely appropriate care	Mild claudication (RC 1) with one-, two-, or three-vessel IP disease
	Moderate–severe (RC 2–3) claudication symptoms with one-vessel IP disease
	Major tissue loss (RC 6) with one-vessel IP disease

Table 5.2 The infrapopliteal lesion severity classification based on the Trans-Atlantic Inter-Society Consensus (TASC) group

TASC lesion type	Description
Type A	Single stenoses, 1 cm in the tibial or peroneal vessels
Type B	Multiple focal stenoses of the tibial or peroneal vessels, each, 1 cm in length
	One or two focal stenoses, each, 1 cm long, at the tibial trifurcation
	Short tibial or peroneal stenosis in conjunction with femoropopliteal angioplasty
Type C	Stenoses 1–4 cm in length
	Occlusions 1–2 cm in length of the tibial or peroneal vessels
	Extensive stenoses of the tibial trifurcation
Type D	Tibial or peroneal occlusions >2 cm
	Diffusely diseased tibial or peroneal vessels

endovascular treatment of BTK atherosclerotic disease in the context of moderate to severe claudication. Table 5.1 summarizes the current Society of Cardiovascular Angiography and Intervention (SCAI) recommendations with regard to appropriateness of treatment of infrapopliteal arterial disease [7].

The infrapopliteal lesion severity classification based on the Trans-Atlantic Inter-Society Consensus (TASC) group is summarized in Table 5.2 [8, 9].

Unfortunately, the TASC II recommendations do not provide detailed information on endovascular therapy for BTK lesions [10]. In addition, they fall short of recognizing the diffuse nature of tibial disease. Patients with CLI and wounds require direct in-line blood flow to the ulcer bed – including often the plantar circulation. Traditionally, complex TASC lesions (C and D) including long CTOs (>2 cm) or severely calcified and diffuse disease were the domain of surgical bypass – preferably with an autologous vein conduit. The debate between the two forms of revascularization therapy reflects in part the somewhat counterintuitive relationship between vessel patency and healing. Surgical bypass for BTK disease has superior patency to angioplasty-based endovascular therapy; however limb salvage rates are not significantly different between the two approaches [11, 12]. This finding does not imply that long-term patency is not important, but rather that the goal of wound healing can generally be achieved within 6 months or less following restoration of arterial flow [13].

The comparatively lower morbidity (compared to open surgery) and advent of novel catheter-based techniques and technologies have encouraged many vascular specialists to take an endovascular first approach to BTK disease [14]. There is a paucity of randomized data in this context. The BASIL trial published in 2005 compared angioplasty against surgical bypass in patients largely with CLI, and the results supported the efficacy of a percutaneous approach with reduced morbidity compared to surgery [12, 15, 16]. Longer-term follow-up of the data suggested a mortality benefit in the surgical arm. However, often lost and relevant to this chapter is that at the time of enrollment into the BASIL trial, 34% of patients had anatomy not suitable for surgical or endovascular therapy. With advances in percutaneous techniques including pedal approaches, dedicated wires and crossing devices, atherectomy, and novel balloon catheters, it is conceivable that many "non-treatable" patients in older studies would now be candidates for therapy – particularly for modern endovascular modalities. This hypothesis will be tested, in part, with the ongoing BEST-CLI study [17].

5.3   BTK CTOs: Prevalence, Angiosome Concept, and Pathology

Any endovascular specialist treating patients with CLI will become intimately familiar with CTOs. The prevalence of BTK CTOs in patients with CLI is 60–70%, and these occlusions are often coupled with multilevel disease (50–60%) [18]. The most common vessels which are occluded are the anterior and posterior tibial arteries – with frequent sparing of the peroneal artery [19]. When evaluating BTK disease – particularly CTOs by angiography – it is imperative to obtain high-quality digital subtraction images. For this purpose, once above-the-knee (ATK) circulation is evaluated, a catheter placed in the popliteal artery with injection of the BTK vessels in orthogonal views is crucial. The imaging of the CTO stump, any "islands" of contrast filling, the distal reconstitution, and status of the dorsal and plantar arches (Fig. 5.2) are fundamental and may require selective cannulation of the individual tibial vessels. We often use a long (150 cm) 0.035/0.038″ diameter support catheter for this purpose and administer intra-arterial nitroglycerin prior to injections. It is important to note that often injection through a retrograde sheath will provide imaging of a vessel lumen which was not visible through antegrade contrast delivery

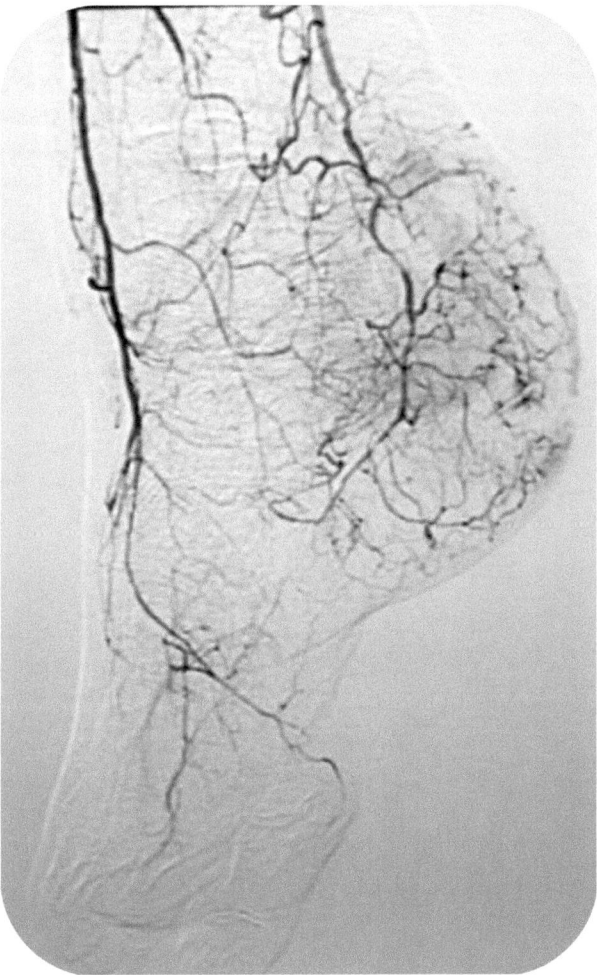

Fig. 5.2 Digital subtraction image of the pedal plantar circulation. Note the diffuse disease of the posterior tibial artery, calcaneal branches, and dorsalis pedis arteries. The plantar circulation is interrupted

(Fig. 5.3a, b). In this regard, simultaneous antegrade and retrograde injections can also help define the CTO length and path.

Although perhaps less certain in the context of surgical bypass, the improved outcomes with endovascular therapy over the past decade have been in part due to a better understanding of the angiosome concept [20]. When evaluating BTK CTOs, the vessel targets for therapy should be evaluated in the context of the angiosome most likely to result in healing of the ulcer (Fig. 5.4). While indirect therapy is often employed due to patient anatomy, a direct angiosome-based revascularization is associated with improved limb salvage [21]. Failure of angiosome-directed therapy for BTK CTOs can be multifactorial and include a poorly defined proximal or distal cap, lack of pedal vessels for retrograde access, and heavy calcification.

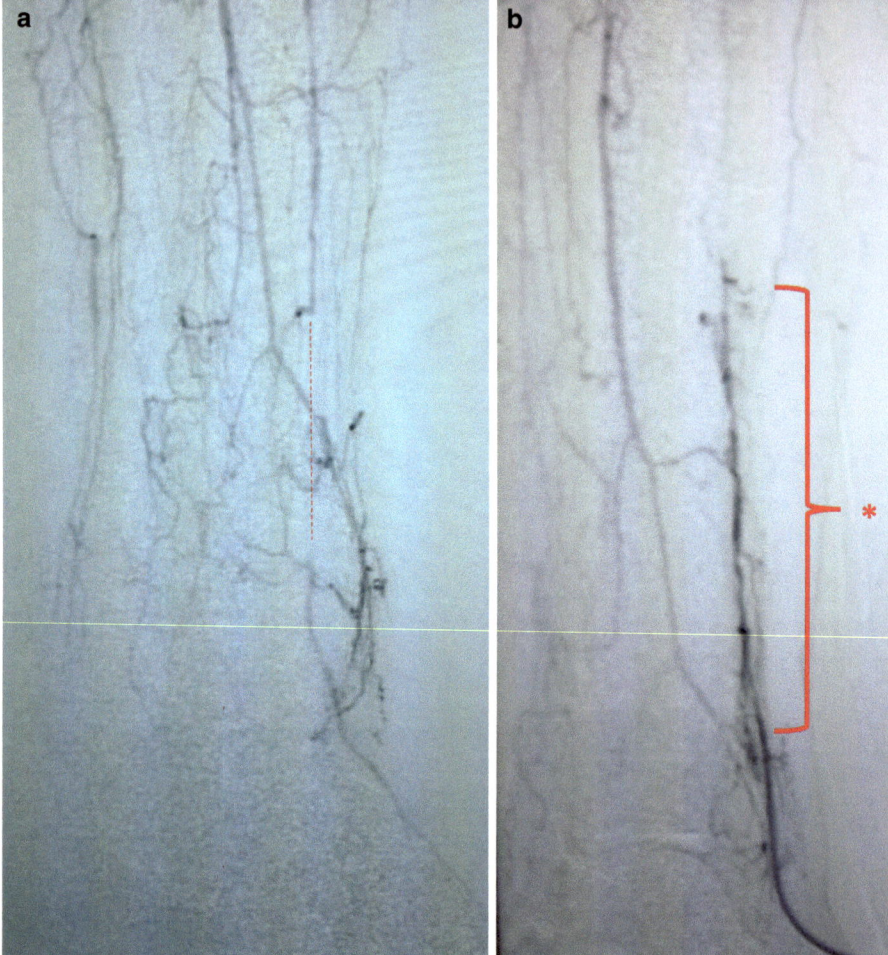

Fig. 5.3 (**a**) Digital subtraction image of the distal anterior tibial CTO (*dashed line*). Image obtained from antegrade injection. (**b**) Magnified image of same patient with retrograde injection through 4 Fr sheath in the dorsalis pedis. Hibernating vessel lumen now visible with retrograde injection (*)

The histopathology of BTK CTOs has important clinical ramifications and therefore warrants some mention. Calcification and diffuse disease – both signatures of BTK CTOs – are common in diabetic patients and in those with chronic renal failure. Fluoroscopically, it may be challenging to distinguish medial (Monckeberg's calcification) from calcification involving luminal compromise. Both pathologic studies and optical coherence tomography (OCT) studies of vessels taken from amputated limbs have provided insight into the role of calcification [22]. As shown in Fig. 5.5, BTK CTOs may have extensive circumferential calcification with compression of the true lumen. This calcium deposition, in part, explains the rationale

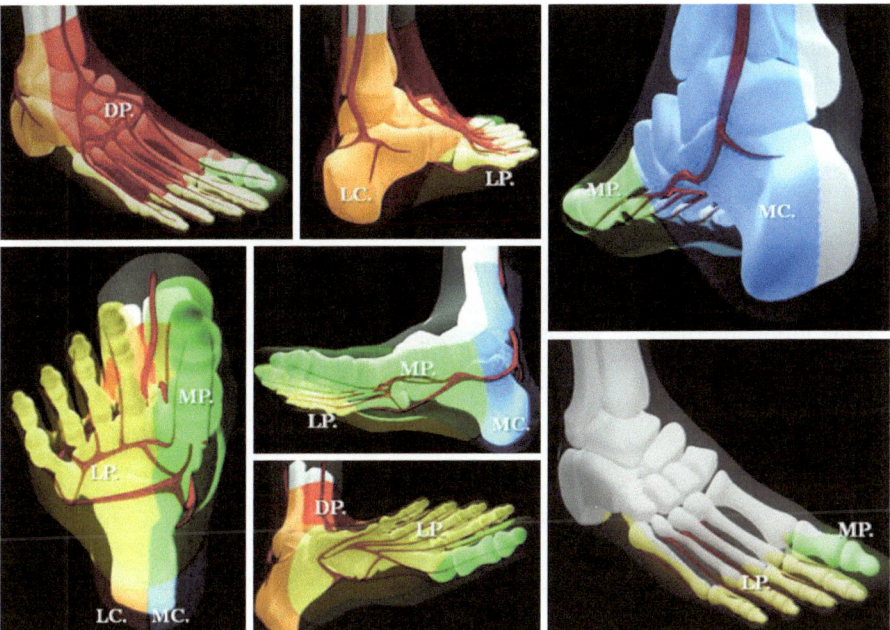

Fig. 5.4 Angiosomes of the foot. *DP* dorsalis pedis artery angiosome, *LP* lateral plantar artery angiosome, *MP* medial plantar artery angiosome, *LC* lateral calcaneal artery angiosome, *MC* medial calcaneal artery angiosome (From: Alexandrescu and Hubermont [20])

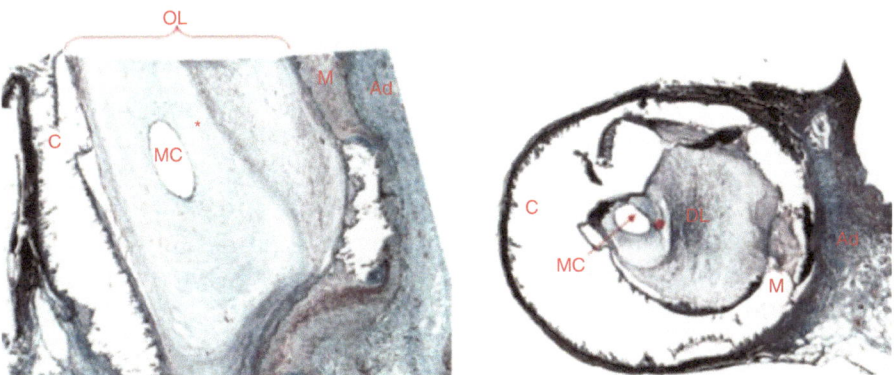

Fig. 5.5 Histologic cross sections of a heavily calcified below-the-knee CTO vessel. *MC* Microchannels, *C* extensive calcification, *OL* occluded lumen, *M* media, *Ad* adventitia. The (*) identifies an area of less dense tissue (collagen) surrounding the microchannel (From: Munce et al. [22])

for atherectomy techniques to modify vessel compliance prior to angioplasty. Beyond the proximal cap and cranial to the distal cap, microchannel(s) may exist which are the endovascular targets of wire navigation. The true lumen surrounding these microchannels has extensive lipid deposition and fibrosis with deposition of smooth muscle cells and collagen. Less commonly thrombus – often organized and surrounding the microchannels – may be present in the lumen of the BTK CTO.

5.4 BTK CTOs: Endovascular Approach

When a decision has been made to attempt endovascular therapy of a BTK CTO, the case should be well planned out. The approach to the procedure can be summarized in the following steps: access, crossing strategy, reentry, and treatment strategy.

5.4.1 Access

5.4.1.1 Access: Contralateral

The most common approach used to treat infrainguinal PAD remains contralateral femoral access. While this access is comfortable to most operators and suitable for many ATK lesions, several issues may arise when treating BTK CTOs using this approach. Some of these concerns include sheath support for calcified lesions, balloon and device length relative to patient height, and concerns over image quality and excessive contrast use. If contralateral access is to be used, then a longer 55, 65, or >70 cm sheath is reasonable. When coupled with adequate anticoagulation (ACT >200 s) and intact inflow, the use of long contralateral sheaths in our experience has been safe – even when placed across the profunda femoris artery.

5.4.1.2 Access: Antegrade

Antegrade access provides many advantages over the contralateral approach including substantially increased device support, ability to access distal vessels, and excellent image quality. Traditionally, antegrade access was cumbersome and challenging. With the use of ultrasound (US)-guided micropuncture cannulation, access success can be improved greatly. Patient and operator comfort should be maximized during antegrade access. Depending on the mobility of the imaging equipment and radiation protection shields, the patient can be placed in a reversed supine position with the feet under the flat panel and the head covered with a raised drape ("tent") to minimize claustrophobia. Our experience has found that medial angulation of the micropuncture needle avoids bias into the profunda femoral artery and is more likely to allow wire delivery to the superficial femoral artery (SFA). If the micropuncture wire favors the profunda and entry is at or above the common femoral bifurcation, then a small microsheath can be placed into the profunda with the wire kept in place. A second angled hydrophilic wire (e.g., V18 Control Wire, Boston

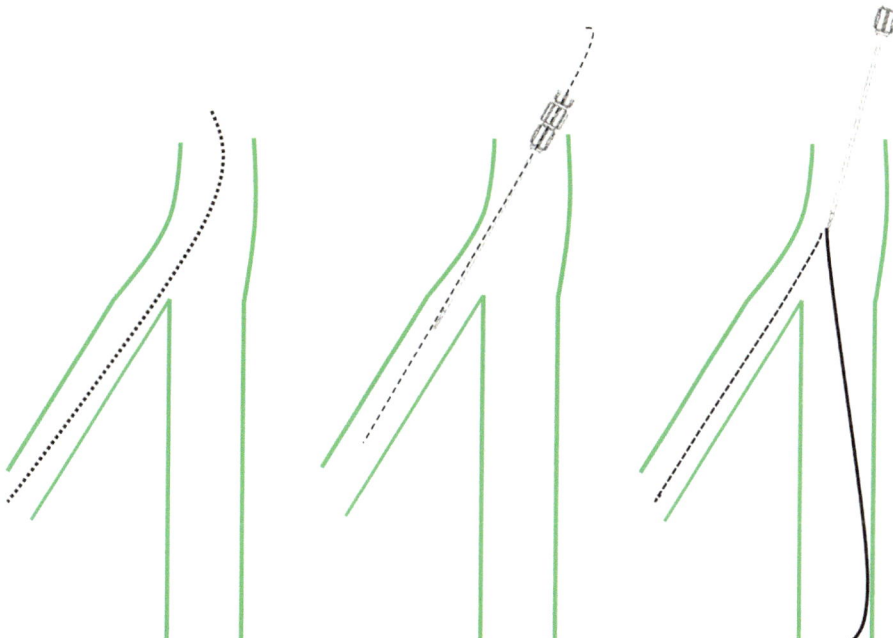

Fig. 5.6 Steps for antegrade access using the profunda femoris for support. (**a**) Micro-wire in place in the profunda. (**b**) Sheath advanced on micro-wire. (**c**) Second hydrophilic wire advanced into superficial femoral artery with the sheath retracted to the bifurcation

Scientific, Marlborough, MA) can then be used to wire the SFA as the sheath is withdrawn back to the bifurcation (Fig. 5.6). The sheath with micro-dilator support is then advanced over the V18 into the SFA and then exchanged for a larger sheath. In general the use of a stiff 0.035″ guidewire (Amplatz Super Stiff, Boston Scientific) for support during sheath placement is helpful with the pannus retracted back by a second operator or assistant. Although access is usually preferred in the common femoral artery where compression can be achieved with manual pressure, access at the junction of the CFA and SFA or even in the first cm of the SFA is acceptable and lowers the risk of retroperitoneal bleeding. However, more distal access of the SFA should be avoided due to the risk of bleeding into the thigh and potential for compartment syndrome. With the increased availability of extravascular closure devices (e.g., Mynx, AccessClosure, Inc., Santa Clara, CA), closure of antegrade access – even involving SFA entry – should be strongly considered.

5.4.1.3   Access: Retrograde Pedal Access

The option of retrograde pedal or distal tibial access should be considered when planning a BTK CTO intervention, and comfort with this technique can increase procedural success [23]. The rationale underlying retrograde access mirrors that of

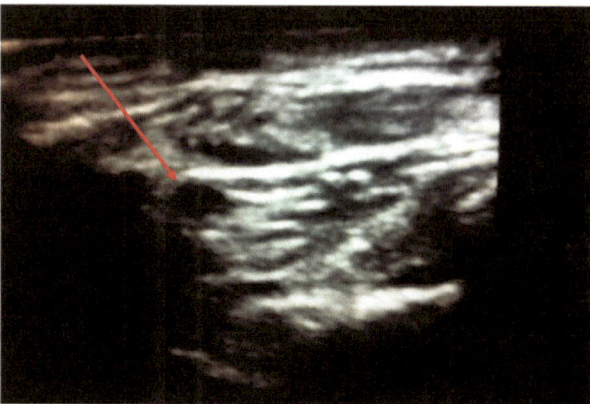

Fig. 5.7 Ultrasound image of the dorsalis pedis artery. *Arrow* indicates vessel target

the CTO approach in the coronary circulation. The proximal caps of BTK CTOs may not always be well defined or may be associated with a proximal collaterals which can bias wires. The distal caps of BTK CTOs may in some cases be less resistant to penetration as compared to proximal caps. Microchannels and vessel islands may not be readily apparent with antegrade injection but can be seen with retrograde injection as discussed earlier.

Visualization options for access include use of fluoroscopic landmarks coupled with angiography or direct ultrasound-guided micropuncture. With the availability of ultrasound-visible needles and handheld ultrasound systems, we recommend this latter approach. The ultrasound scan of the target vessel should ideally be performed with a high-frequency (7–15 MHz) hockey stick probe (Fig. 5.7). Vessel diameter (ideally ≥2 mm), degree of calcification, and tortuosity should be evaluated. If possible, the access point should be sufficiently distal as to allow the sheath tip to be several mm proximal to the distal cap. Common sites for access include the dorsalis pedis, the PT just above the medial malleolus, and the distal AT above the ankle. More challenging is access of the peroneal artery due to its deeper course and concerns with hemostasis. Despite these issues, the peroneal artery can be accessed, and awareness of potential bleeding should be kept in mind coupled with the availability of coronary diameter covered stents should hemostasis fail. Entry into the artery can be facilitated if the foot is dorsiflexed and rotated out for the posterior tibial and plantar flexed for the dorsalis pedis artery. The use of ultrasound also helps inadvertent cannulation of the tibial veins. The flow in the distal tibial arteries in CLI patients is often sluggish; therefore arterial "flash back" can be relatively "venous-like." The ultrasound relationship of the veins and arteries is reliable in that a tibial artery is surrounded by one or more (often 2–3) veins in and the artery is often calcified. The ultrasound probe should be rotated as necessary to see the tip of the microneedle during access, and often steady slow pressure by the needle tip on the arterial wall is required to penetrate the calcium and avoid rolling of the vessel. Much like radial artery access, the use of excessive lidocaine should be avoided, and use of systemic or intra-arterial nitrates can be helpful to minimize spasm.

If the distal anatomic target is poor, retrograde access can still be considered and a micro-dilator only strategy for stability can be used. This type of access is primarily used for retrograde wire passage. Preferably, the placement of a sheath allows for secure access, easier interchange of wires and support catheters, and facilitates angiography. Examples of available sheaths for pedal access include the Cook Micropuncture Pedal Introducer Access Sheath (Cook Medical, Bloomington, IN), (2.9 Fr inner diameter) and the Terumo Pinnacle Precision Access System Sheath (Terumo IS, Somerset, NJ). The latter sheath has a true 4 Fr inner diameter and allows for larger device passage. Once the sheath is in place, copious use of intra-arterial vasodilators including nitroglycerin and calcium channel blockers is paramount. We recommend fairly aggressive anticoagulation once the pedal sheath is in place with ACTs ≥ 250 s. The sheath should be flushed regularly and secured with tape or a clear adhesive covering. Removal of the sheath can be done with manual pressure or use of a radial artery compression band for ankle level access. Hemostasis can generally be achieved, even in the context of an elevated ACT if manual pressure is used. The timing of sheath removal varies upon the procedural approach. If the retrograde access results in successful wire passage across the CTO and the wire is snared from above and externalized with plans for antegrade treatment, then the sheath can be removed prior to conclusion of the intervention with close observation of the pedal access site. It is also helpful to keep in mind that if after successful treatment the flow in the target tibial vessel appears sluggish, the presence of an indwelling distal sheath is a likely cause and the flow should be reevaluated with the sheath pulled out.

5.4.1.4 Access (and Treatment): Tibio-pedal Arterial Minimally Invasive Retrograde Revascularization (TAMI)

Pioneered by Mustapha, Saab and colleagues, the tibio-pedal arterial minimally invasive retrograde revascularization (TAMI) approach is a retrograde pedal or tibial access technique for treatment of BTK disease (and in some cases more proximal disease) [24]. The rationale behind the TAMI approach is to avoid femoral access (either contralateral or antegrade ipsilateral) and therefore avoid the potential for groin site complications, to improve crossing support and to allow for better distal tibial vessel angiographic visualization. Access, pretreatment angiography, treatment, and post-angiography in this technique is done exclusively through the retrograde access. Recently, there has been new equipment developed to deliver therapy in the tibial and plantar circulation. The TAMI technique capitalizes on the ability to deliver different types of balloons, atherectomy, and stenting options via a single pedal sheath. The recent release of the slender sheaths (Terumo), 4/5 Fr, 5/6 Fr, 6/7 Fr, allows for multiple options of revascularization. Atherectomy devices that can be placed though the 4/5 Fr access include orbital atherectomy (CSI Micro crowns 1.25, 1.25 solid, and 1.5 solid) and laser atherectomy up to 1.7 mm catheter. Stent options that can fit through the 4/5 Fr sheaths include the Abbott Xpert stents platform and the non-drug-eluting Zilver stents (Cook Medical). It should be noted that this is a rapidly evolving area, and equipment compatibility with pedal access sheaths is expected to increase in the near future.

Paramount to the TAMI technique is maintenance of the patency of the pedal access vessel. Infusion of a carefully de-aired heparinized vasodilator solution (TAMI solution) into the side arm of the sheath helps prevent vasospasm or thrombosis. This solution consists of 3000 μg nitroglycerin and 2.5–5 mg verapamil mixed with 500 ml of heparinized saline and infused into the arterial sheath at a rate of 6–7 ml/min. The rate can be adjusted depending on the patient's hemodynamics.

Posttreatment imaging is done by placement of a small diameter catheter in the proximal treated vessel connected to a Tuohy-Borst or Copilot system-type connection (Abbott Vascular, Santa Clara, CA) to maintain wire access and allow for injection. The TAMI technique has some drawbacks which warrant mention. It is limited for multilevel disease treatment, cannot be used with directional atherectomy devices (TurboHawk/Silverhawk, Medtronic, Minneapolis, MN) which require antegrade directional cutting, and is best suited for treatment following true lumen passage of the wire. In addition, filter embolic protection devices (EPDs) cannot be used in the TAMI technique, although the presence and aspiration of the sheath in the distal vessel may in theory provide protection to the foot vasculature obviating need for an EPD.

5.4.1.5   Access: Metatarsal and Direct Pedal Loop

An intact pedal loop significantly aids in wound healing, and reconstruction of the distal foot circulation can be approached in multiple ways. Direct access of arch/pedal loop vessels is an option for retrograde recanalization – particularly when antegrade attempts have failed. This access is typically performed in concert with ipsilateral antegrade access. Access of the pedal loop has been pioneered by Palena and colleagues [25, 26]. Access into the pedal loop circulation is often best achieved with puncture of the first dorsal metatarsal artery; alternatively direct access of the loop itself may be considered (Fig. 5.8a, b). Given the small size of these vessels, use of careful fluoroscopic or ultrasound-guided landmarks (calcification) to guide access with copious pretreatment with vasodilators is key. Access is obtained with a 21 gauge microneedle and a microsheath is placed (Cook sheath, Cook Medical, Bloomington, IN). It is not necessary or even possible in many cases to place the entire length of the sheath in the access vessel – rather once the sheath is several

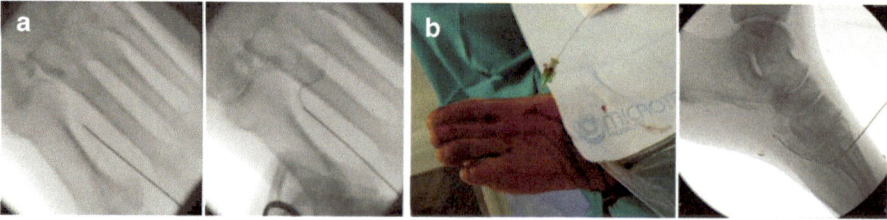

Fig. 5.8 Metatarsal access (**a**) and pedal plantar loop access (**b**) (From: Manzi and Palena [48])

millimeters in place, it can be secured to the foot with adhesive tape or transparent film. Retrograde crossing can then be performed with 0.014″ or 0.018″ diameter wires with crossing catheter support, with wire capture and treatment from the antegrade approach. The access site sheath can be removed with manual pressure held or alternatively use of a small diameter (2.0 mm) balloon for tamponade. Again given the size of the vessels involved, this approach which remains technically challenging is thus far limited to select centers. Palena and colleagues have noted an acute technical success rate of over 84% without major procedural complications.

5.4.1.6 Access: Radial

There is an increasing interest in use of radial access for angiography and intervention in patients with lower extremity PAD. Intervention thus far has been limited to iliac and femoropopliteal disease, and at this time there is little role of radial in the therapy of BTK disease [27]. Nonetheless long peripheral catheters (e.g., 150 cm, 4 Fr Terumo PV catheter) are available and in shorter patients may provide a means for obtaining diagnostic data if needed.

5.5 Crossing Approach

The choice of access, crossing approach, and treatment strategies are all interrelated. An understanding of catheter and device (balloon, stent, atherectomy catheter, EPD) sizes and sheath compatibility is crucial to successful treatment of BTK CTOs. Bailout strategies if one approach fails should be preplanned. Algorithmic approaches to peripheral CTOs remain in development and as of yet are not as robust as those for coronary CTOs [28]. The two broad approaches are a wire/support catheter technique versus a crossing device strategy. There are data which would suggest that crossing devices may have superior technical success as an initial strategy compared to a wire-based approach in infrainguinal CTOs [29]. Over the past decade, there has been an increase in the availability of crossing devices; however there are no randomized data at this time to support one approach over another in the BTK circulation. In addition the (non-reimbursed) cost of these tools must be taken account when gauging their overall utility in the healthcare system. A summary of current crossing tools is shown in Table 5.3.

Wire strategies have primarily revolved around use of coronary guidewires (3 to 12+ g tip weight) or heavier peripheral specific wires (18 to > 20 g tip weights in either 0.014″ or 0.018″ diameters). Table 5.4 outlines selected wires for BTK CTOs.

Hydrophilic polymer-coated wires can be considered when a microchannel is seen or suspected by angiography. Whether a wire escalation strategy or use of specific wires upfront is the superior method remains unclear, but in general heavily calcified vessels require heavier tip weights. Whether using a crossing device or wire approach, true lumen passage is attractive in the BTK for a number of reasons.

Table 5.3 Selected crossing devices and descriptions

Crossing device	Manufacturer	Description
Viance	Covidien/Medtronic	Blunt manual probing/controlled dissection Can be used retrograde
WildCat/KittyCat	Avinger	Manual or assisted blunt dissection
Ocelot	Avinger	Manual or assisted blunt dissection with OCT guidance
Peripheral Crosser	Bard	High-frequency vibrations to penetrate tissue
TruePath	Boston Scientific	Diamond-coated rapidly rotating tip
Frontrunner XP	Cordis	Blunt microdissection

Table 5.4 Selected wires and characteristics

Wire	Manufacturer	Characteristics
MiracleBros Wires, 0.14″	Abbott/Asahi	3–12 g tip weight Hydrophobic coated
Approach, 0.014″	Cook	6–25 g tip weight PTFE coated
Treasure 12, 0.018″	Asahi	12 g tip weight Hydrophilic tip coating PTFE shaft coating
Astato 30, 0.018″	Asahi	30 g tip weight Hydrophilic tip coating PTFE shaft coating
Astato XS 20, 0.014″	Asahi	20 g tip load Hydrophilic tip coating PTFE shaft coating

True lumen passage allows for potentially more aggressive debulking with atherectomy and avoids the use of stenting. As compared to the SFA bed, the data for infrapopliteal subintimal angioplasty are less robust, though several reports suggest adequate clinical outcomes [30]. Certainly, long areas of subintimal passage can result in impaired flow and often require adjuvant therapy with stents. The small diameter and long length of BTK vessels also limit the choice of available stent technology. General options to deal with subintimal wire or device passage are to attempt reentry or use opposite direction access.

5.5.1 Reentry

True lumen reentry can be challenging – again due to vessel size and calcification. Reentry can be achieved with the use of a stiff angled wire and catheter method to puncture into the true lumen, a needle-based technology such as the Outback (Cordis, Fremont, CA) catheter system or a balloon orientation/penetration wire

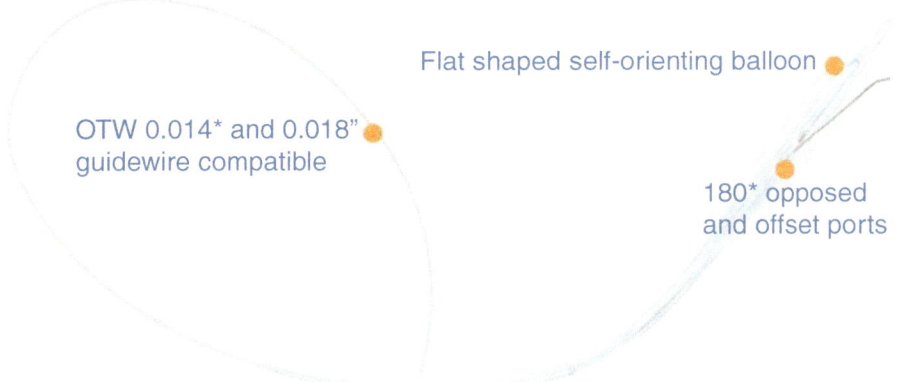

Flat shaped self-orienting balloon

OTW 0.014* and 0.018"
guidewire compatible

180* opposed
and offset ports

Fig. 5.9 Enteer reentry system. The flat-shaped balloon is inflated with 1–2 atm and reorients itself in the subintimal space. A specific Enteer wire (stiff or standard) is advanced through the balloon and is used to puncture into the true lumen

combination such as the Enteer (Medtronic) system (Fig. 5.9). The small profile of this latter tool is particularly helpful at distal reentry in the tibial vessels; an example of use of this device is shown in Fig. 5.10. The technique recommended is to advance the Enteer balloon over the subintimal wire adjacent to the reconstituted vessel. Although the balloon may appear adjacent to the true vessel, orthogonal angulated views should be performed to confirm the position. When inflated the Enteer balloon should lay out in a long cylindrical appearance – generally no more than 1–3 atm are needed to inflate the balloon. The subintimal wire can then be removed and the micro-tapered Enteer wire (either stiff or standard) can be advanced. Manipulation with a torque device should be performed of the Enteer wire such that it exits the balloon through the side port directed toward the target vessel. We have generally found that the standard wire below the knee is sufficient for reentry – with the stiff wire reserved for above the knee or heavily calcified tibial vessel use. Gentle but steady focused pressure is often required to puncture the true lumen in cases of calcification. Once the Enteer wire has entered the true lumen, it should be freely mobile. Given the "needle-like" nature of this wire, it should not be advanced far distally – rather the balloon should be deflated, removed, and the Enteer wire exchanged for a workhorse wire. Generally, avoidance of heavily calcified segments is recommended for selection of a reentry zone.

5.5.2   *Opposite Direction Wire Strategies*

It is our preference to stay true luminal or at least keep the length of subintimal passage to a minimum for BTK CTO recanalization and therefore allow for adjunctive atherectomy. The use of intravascular ultrasound can be helpful to determine the

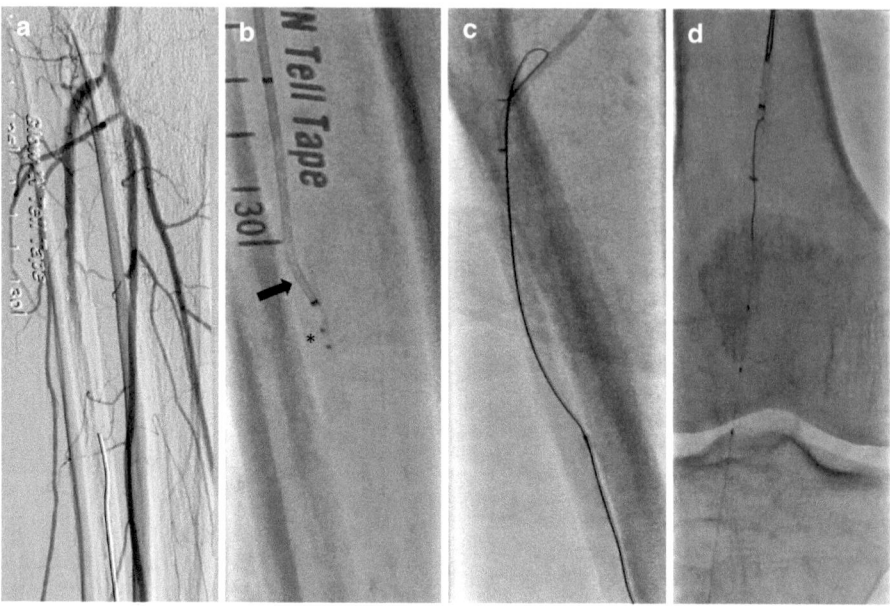

Fig. 5.10 Anterior tibial CTO. (**a**) A retrograde wire has entered into the subintimal space. (**b**) The Enteer catheter (*) is advanced through the retrograde sheath. An antegrade catheter (*arrow*) marks the true lumen. (**c**) Once the wire is in the true lumen, it is exchanged for a workhorse wire and advanced. (**d**) The wire is snared and brought into the antegrade sheath

extent of subintimal passage, location of true lumen exit, and select segments which can be treated with atherectomy. If a wire (or catheter) strategy results in entry into the subintimal space (either from an antegrade or retrograde approach) and device-assisted reentry is not used (or fails), then passage of a second wire in the opposite direction can be attempted. The goal of this second wire is true lumen passage when possible, but if not, a variety of subintimal space strategies including controlled antegrade and retrograde tracking and dissection (CART) and subintimal arterial flossing with antegrade-retrograde intervention (SAFARI) techniques can be considered. The CART technique involves inflation of a small diameter (2.0 mm) over the retrograde wire while trying to advance the antegrade wire located in the subintimal space into the true distal lumen. Reverse CART is the same technique with reversal of the balloon inflation onto the antegrade wire when the retrograde wire has entered the subintimal space (Fig. 5.11). The SAFARI technique has been described in the tibial vessels, and akin to the knuckle technique in coronary CTOs involves intentional entry into the subintimal space [30]. This entry is facilitated by generating a looped tip on the guidewire and dissecting past the occluded segment to join the subintimal space from an opposite wire. The entry into the subintimal space on both ends is dilated with a balloon or catheter prior to definitive angioplasty. Though the data are relatively scarce, this technique is associated with an adequate technical success rates (70–80%); however given technological advancements in true lumen crossing tools and reentry devices, the SAFARI technique is less commonly used in contemporary practice.

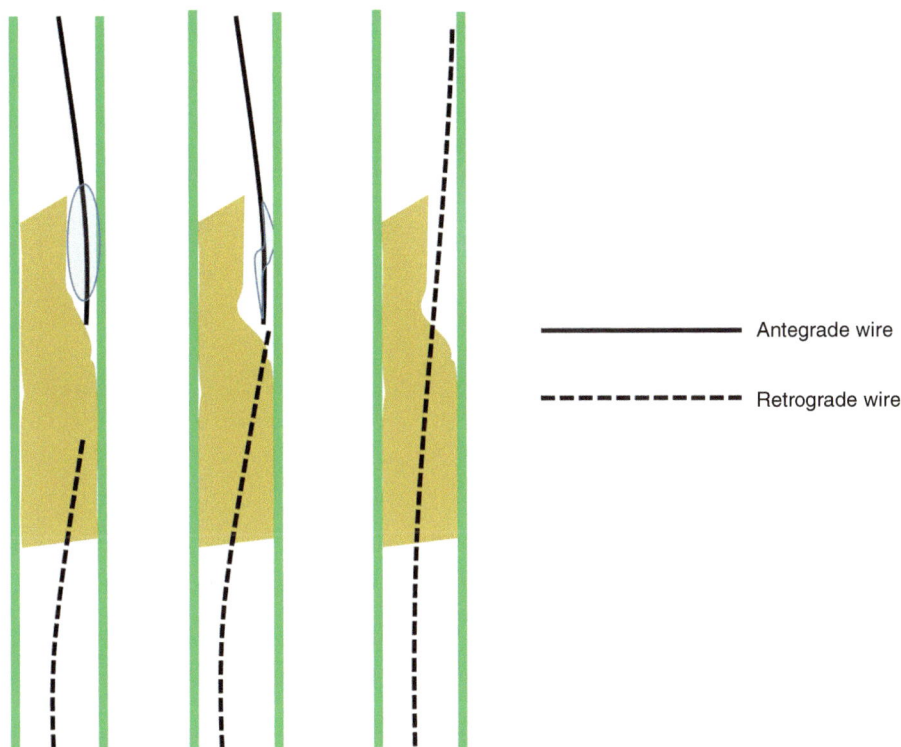

Fig. 5.11 Reverse CART. Angioplasty over antegrade wire creates a space for advancement of the retrograde wire

5.5.3 *Wire Capture*

If retrograde techniques will be used and antegrade treatment performed, then wire capture will be required during the case (Fig. 5.12). The simplest (and most cost-effective) method is to directly wire the antegrade sheath. Generally this is facilitated by a small loop at the tip of the wire and prolapse into the sheath. Alternatively if a Viance catheter is used, this catheter when spun generally enters the sheath without difficulty. Rarely, 2 mm diameter snares (or multi-loop gooseneck snares) can be used to externalize wires. The superficial femoral artery allows for the easiest deployment of snares without risk of injury to the smaller BTK vessels. In our experience, snaring wires – particularly 0.014 or 0.018″ diameters – requires some time and patience. An alternative device is the Quick-Cross Capture catheter (Spectranetics, Colorado Springs, CO), which is a balloon-supported funnel-shaped wire capture device. Inflation of the balloon centers the funnel in the middle of the vessel (generally used in the SFA), and the wire then has limited options but to enter the funnel. Once in the device it is advanced through the length of the catheter and easily externalized. When not using such a device or a snare, externalization of the

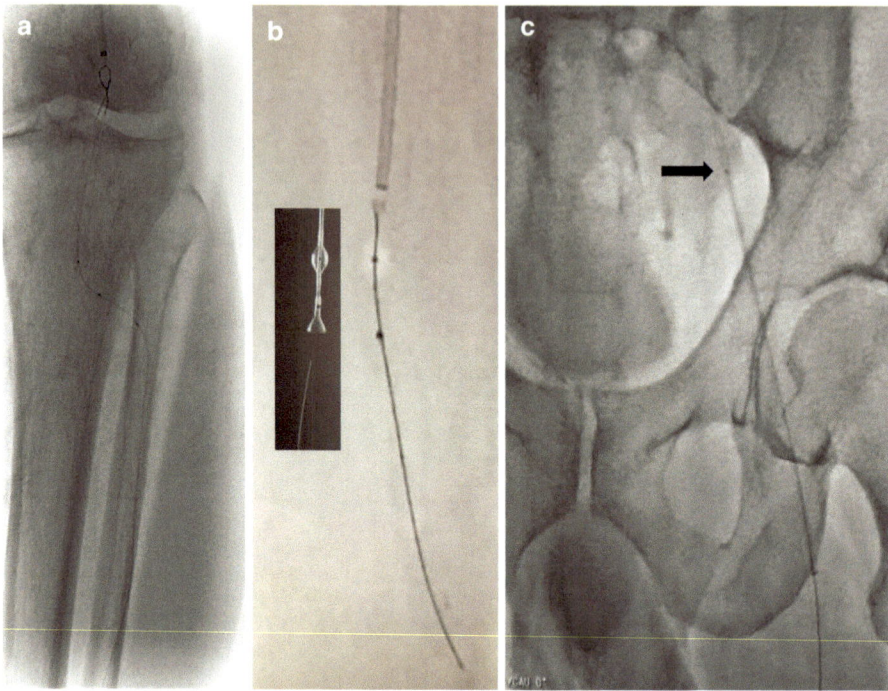

Fig. 5.12 Wire capture without snares. (**a**) A retrograde wire is advanced into the sheath. A loop on the tip helps to "knuckle" the wire into the sheath. (**b**) A Spectranetics (Colorado Springs, CO) Quick-Cross Capture catheter is advanced through the antegrade sheath. This catheter has a balloon that when inflated centers the lumen of the catheter to the vessel. A funnel (see *insert*) at the distal end of the catheter directs the wire into the lumen. (**c**) A Viance catheter (Medtronic) (*arrow*) is advanced retrograde from a pedal sheath into the common femoral artery where it is directed into the sheath by rapid torque delivery

wire can be challenging as the sheath hub must be removed and the wire pulled out. This process may lead to blood loss from the sheath and reattachment of the hub over the floppy end of the guidewire may be challenging. To minimize this issue, a 90 cm 0.035″ support catheter can be inserted into the sheath and the guidewire advanced through the tip of the catheter and out of the sheath (Fig. 5.13).

5.5.4 Extravascular Ultrasound-Guided Crossing (EVUS)

The concept of using extravascular ultrasound-guided crossing (EVUS) represents the natural evolution of using US in the endovascular lab. Traditionally, the use of US has been reserved for obtaining access in vascular conduits including arteries and veins. The use of US in obtaining access for variety of vessels has been examined by Mustapha, Saab et al. and has been shown to be safe and effective in obtaining access across all vascular beds including tibial/plantar circulation [31].

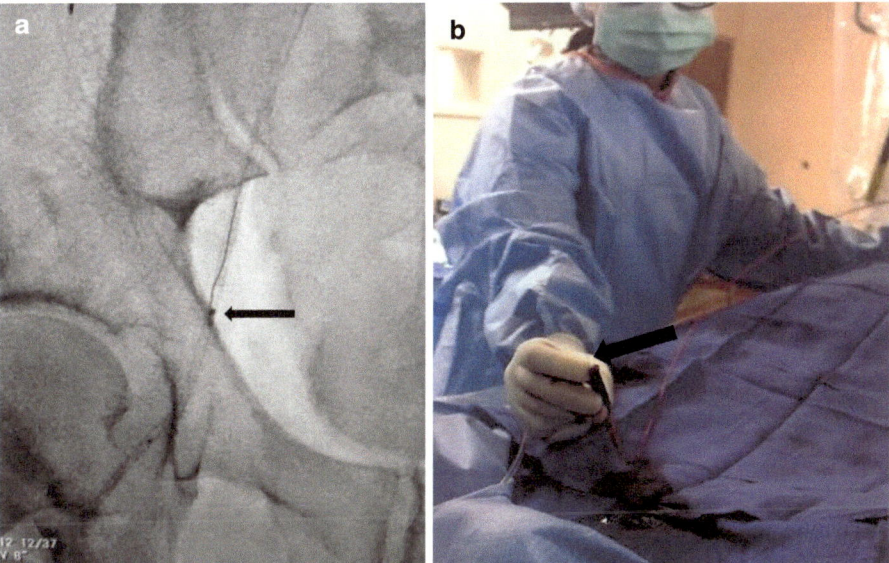

Fig. 5.13 Wire externalization without snare. (**a**) A retrograde 0.014" wire is advanced into the contralateral sheath and fed into a 90 cm 0.035" support catheter (*arrow*). (**b**) The wire is then externalized (*arrow*) through the support catheter without need to manipulate the sheath hub

Fig. 5.14 Retrograde tibial wire deflected to subintimal plane by the tibial CTO

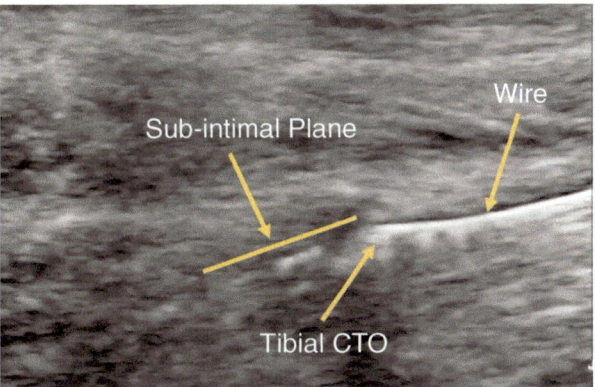

EVUS allows the operator to visualize wires, CTO crossing tools, catheters, atherectomy, and stenting devices and to direct their equipment in real time. Direct visualization is particularly important as the operator is attempting to cross a CTO. Knowing when the wire goes into a subintimal plane or extravascular space has important implications on treatment decisions and options. Figure 5.14 shows a retrograde CTO wire crossing from the true lumen into the subintimal plane. This is a critical stage in the procedure as the operator may choose to obtain alternative access or may consider the use of reentry devices. Furthermore, one may make the argument that the EVUS approach may increase the safety of the procedure by reducing radiation and the amount of contrast.

5.6 Treatment Strategies

5.6.1 Balloon Angioplasty

Percutaneous transluminal angioplasty (PTA) remains the mainstay of treatment for BTK CTOs. Evaluation in balloon technology has resulted in improved crossing profiles, longer shaft, and balloon lengths. In addition, tapered balloons are available which help approximate the natural size changes of tibial vessels [32]. In addition to 0.014″ dedicated peripheral balloons, coronary balloons are frequently used in the treatment of BTK disease and particularly in distal vessels which have improved crossing ability as compared to their peripheral counterparts. Focal PTA is often necessary at fibrotic or calcific spots prior to delivery of longer peripheral balloons. The technique for PTA is similar to other vascular beds where a methodical gradual inflation at a 1:1 vessel to balloon ratio for several minutes (3–5 min) followed by slow deflation is recommended. Dissections are not uncommon but with attention to technique, rarely flow limiting. With the concern for dissections and the fibro-calcific nature of BTK plaque, there has been significant interest in specialty balloons designed to score plaque or prevent intimal damage (Table 5.5). Limited data would suggest that these balloons may result in fewer dissections, but long-term efficacy data compared to traditional angioplasty is lacking. Apart from dissections, the drawbacks of PTA are elastic recoil and neointimal hyperplasia. In selected studies, the primary patency rates with PTA have been reported as low as 40–50% range at 1 year, while other data would suggest patency rates up to 70% in shorter lesions. However it should be kept in mind that wound healing rates, as discussed above, with PTA only approach are comparable to surgical bypass – despite higher restenosis. If a PTA approach is taken and there is stalled healing, restenosis should be considered and the threshold for repeat angiography and intervention kept low.

Table 5.5 Specialty balloons for BTK angioplasty

Balloon	Manufacturer	Description
Flextome Cutting Balloon	Boston Scientific	Noncompliant balloon with blades which score plaque
AngioSculpt	Spectranetics	Helical nitinol scoring elements modify plaque
Chocolate	TriReme	Semi-compliant balloon in a nitinol cage which distributes inflation forces along the balloon limiting risk of dissection

5.6.2 Bare Metal Stents

The role of stenting for BTK disease has primarily been to treat flow-limiting dissections or persistent elastic recoil. The relative smaller diameter of the tibial vessels, coupled with their length, and often impaired outflow limit the role of extensive stenting. The choices for bare metal stents include 2.0–4.0 coronary balloon expandable stents or 3.0–4.0 nitinol self-expanding stents (Xpert stents, Abbot vascular). When balloon expandable stents are used in the context of CLI, the primary patency and freedom from target lesion revascularization rates range between 50–70%. Nitinol self-expanding stents were studied by Rocha Singh et al. in the XCELL trial [13]. The 6-month binary restenosis rate approached 70%, with clinically driven freedom from TLR rate of 70.1% at 12 months and 1-year wound healing rates of 54.4%. Though generally felt to be effective, these data in total suggest that bare metal stenting is modestly better than PTA alone and highlight the challenges with BTK vessel patency.

5.6.3 Drug-Eluting Technologies

Potentially, mitigating the impact of restenosis is delivery of anti-smooth muscle proliferation therapy either by way of drug-eluting stents (DES) or drug-coated (primarily paclitaxel) balloons. DES available widely for over a decade for the coronary arteries have been studied in the BTK circulation. Single-center studies and registries have demonstrated excellent primary patency rates averaging in the 90% range [33]. Randomized data including the YUKON-BTK trial, the ACHILLES trial, and the DESTINY trial demonstrate similar results in terms of patency and freedom from TLR [34]. Despite these data, DES are not a panacea for the treatment of CLI. Limitations include the short lengths of available DES (38 mm currently in the United States) relative to lesion lengths (150–200 mm CTOs are common), cost of placement of multiple DES, potential risk of stent thrombosis with potential need for longer-terms antiplatelet therapy, impairment of landing zones for future bypass, management of no stent zones near the ankle and near tibial plateau, and stents may be a poor choice in many small diameter diffusely diseased vessel. For these reasons, the use of DCB technology has gained much interest. Small pilot trials, including the DEBATE BTK study (Drug-Eluting Balloon in Peripheral Intervention for Below-the-Knee Angioplasty), demonstrated superior patency and lower restenosis rates as compared to standard PTA [35]. A handful of larger trials are currently underway examining the role of drug-coated (paclitaxel) balloons in the tibial circulation. These include the LUTONIX BTK (Lutonix Drug-Coated Balloon Versus Standard Balloon Angioplasty for Treatment of Below-the-Knee Arteries) and the BAIR trial (Paclitaxel-Coated Versus Uncoated Balloon for the Treatment of Below-the-Knee In-Stent Restenosis) [33]. The results of the Medtronic INPACT DEEP trial

(Randomized Study of IN.PACT Amphirion Drug-Eluting Balloon vs Standard PTA for the Treatment of Below-the-Knee Critical Limb Ischemia) were recently published [36]. The study demonstrated no significant benefit in terms of TLR or late lumen loss with DCB as compared to standard PTA. There was a numerical but not statistically significant increase in amputations with DCB therapy. The precise role and method of delivery of anti-restenosis therapy BTK remains to be better defined.

5.6.3.1 Atherectomy

The increase in atherectomy use for the treatment of lower extremity PAD has been profound over the past decade. The availability of choices of therapy from rotational, orbital, directional, and laser has grown tremendously over this period of time. There remains a paucity of data to suggest that one atherectomy device is superior to another in terms of angiographic or clinical endpoints relevant to CLI. Furthermore, the real-world role of atherectomy remains primarily as an adjunctive tool for debulking or vessel modification in concert with PTA. The growth in atherectomy use is likely multifactorial as these devices have allowed interventionists to take on more complex disease – which may have necessitated bypass in the past and allowed improved angiographic results in calcified vessels. It should also be noted that the favorable reimbursement for atherectomy in the United States has no doubt added to the more widespread use and development of atherectomy devices.

Given the lack of large adequately powered randomized studies, considerations of atherectomy device selection should be made based on practical concerns. Several commonly used BTK atherectomy tools are summarized in Table 5.6.

5.7 Complications of BTK CTO Revascularization

As with treatment of any peripheral lesion, there are risks associated with each step of therapy of BTK CTOs. Given that most cases are performed for limb salvage in patients often with multi-organ dysfunction, major procedural complications can significantly reduce the likelihood of wound healing and result in increased morbidity and mortality. Specific complications which warrant discussion include distal embolization and management of vessel perforation.

5.7.1 Distal Embolization

Distal embolization (DE) can take the form of subclinical or clinically relevant events. A potential classification scheme is introduced in the table. Subclinical DE occurs commonly during endovascular therapy and has been detected by Doppler

Table 5.6 Selected atherectomy devices with mode of action and key clinical data

Device	Manufacturer	Mode of action	Key clinical data
CSI	Cardiovascular Systems Incorporated	Orbital atherectomy: diamond-coated crown which rotates at speeds varying from 60,000 to 200,000 rpm Ablates plaque to particle sizes 2 μm [37] Sizing of crowns: **Tibials/peroneal** *Reference vessel diameter:* *2–4 mm* 1.25 mm Solid Crown 1.50 mm Classic Crown 1.25 mm Solid Micro Crown **Below the ankle** *Reference vessel diameter:* *2–4 mm* 1.25 mm Solid Micro Crown Micro crown 1.25 mm size can be used retrograde through 4 Fr precision (Terumo) sheath Treats lesion in both directions Device used over a ViperWire (0.014″ or 0.017″ tipped) Filter rarely needed, but NAV6 filter system (Abbott) can be used off-label by back loading on 0.017″ tipped ViperWire (CSI)	The CONFIRM registry demonstrated that in highly calcified lesions, treatment with CSI atherectomy and adjunctive balloon angioplasty (PTA) was effective with a reduction in stenosis from an average of 88% to about 10%, with a low percentage (5.1%) of bail-out stenting due to dissection [38] The OASIS trial, which focused on infrapopliteal lesions, demonstrated a low dissection rate (2.5%) with a CSI atherectomy + PTA strategy with a 90.1% procedural success rate [38]
Jetstream	Boston Scientific	Rotational atherectomy device with or without blade deployment for additional cutting Atherectomy is coupled with active aspiration of debris JETSTREAM XC (above the knee) and SC (below the knee [BTK], 1.6 mm and 1.85 mm devices) The SC devices do not have expandable blades Device used over a 0.014″ JETWIRE. Off-label use over filter wires has been performed. Care should be taken when using over Spiderwire (Medtronic) to avoid vessel trauma or filter damage from rotation of the filter during atherectomy Minimum sheath size is 7 Fr	Multicenter Pathway PVD trial. Had 210 lesions (18 were BTK). TLR rates at 6 months and 12 months for BTK lesions were 7.7% and 15.4%, respectively [39]

(continued)

Table 5.6 (continued)

Device	Manufacturer	Mode of action	Key clinical data
Laser	Spectranetics	Excimer laser emits energy at a wavelength of 308 nm ablating thrombus and plaque Strengths are for crossing "un-crossable" lesions Most commonly used with adjunctive PTA	The LACI registry examined the role of adjunctive laser atherectomy to PTA or stenting. A 92% limb salvage rate at 6 months was demonstrated [40]
Phoenix	Volcano Corporation	Front cutting system based on the Archimedes screw which captures and delivers plaque to a waste bag 5–6 Fr, 1.8–2.2 mm catheter tip for BTK application	The EASE study was a prospective, multicenter, single-arm study of 105 patients (123 lesions). The majority of lesions were at or below the knee. Reported technical success of 95.1% (Results presented at VIVA 2013)
Rotablator	Boston Scientific	Diamond tipped front cutting burr delivered over a 0.009 burr Can be delivered through a 4 Fr sheath or larger 1.5, 1.75 or 2.0 burr sizes used for BTK applications	150 patients with 212 lesions, 55% of the lesions BTK [41]. 37 complications including perforation, dissection, slow flow were reported. Overall technical success rate with adjuvant PTA was 97%
TurboHawk/ SilverHawk	Medtronic	Directional cutting device with packing of plaque into nose cone Small vessel BTK cutters include SS , SC, and EXL and ES (2–4 mm, 2–3 mm diameter target vessels, respectively), 6 Fr sheath compatible Distal tibial and pedal cutter: DS 1.5–2.0, 5 Fr sheath compatible	The DEFINITIVE LE study enrolled 800 patients with 18.5% lesions overall BTK in a prospective multicenter trial [42]. The study included 201 patients with CLI (34.4% BTK lesions). Procedural success of 83% in the CLI patients, with a 95% freedom from amputation at 12 months

ultrasound studies which note high-intensity signals (HITS) during interventions. Between subclinical and frank clinically relevant DE are more subtle angiographic findings such as small vessel cutoffs or loss of side branches. These events may not have immediate clinical impact or be amenable to further therapy; however their longer-term impact on main vessel patency or limb salvage is unknown. Clinically relevant DE, i.e., events which result in symptoms (pain, tissue loss) or result in macrovascular flow impairment, appears to occur in 1–4% of cases [43]. When a macro-embolus is visible, it may be retrieved using aspiration thrombectomy catheters (see Fig. 5.15) [44, 45]. For more diffuse DE, use of a prolonged

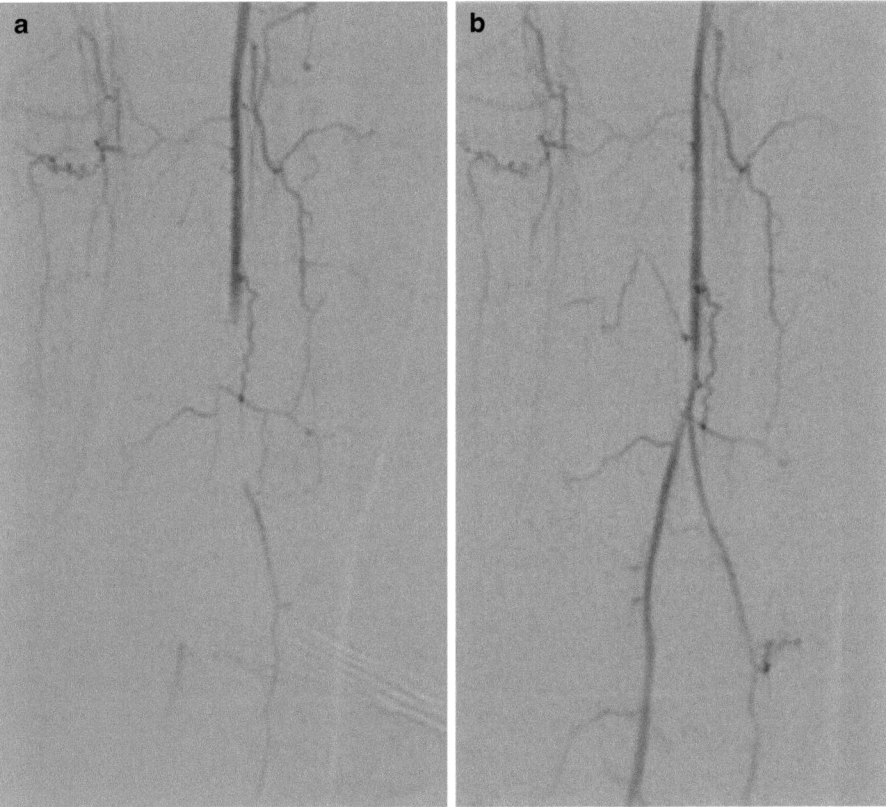

Fig. 5.15 Distal embolization of the anterior tibial artery. (**a**) Vessel cutoff, (**b**) after treatment with manual aspiration thrombectomy

catheter-directed thrombolytic infusion may be helpful [46]. Adjuvant use of potent antiplatelet therapy (glycoprotein 2b/3a receptor inhibitors) has been described [47].

Prevention of DE is a key consideration during BTK therapy. A classification scheme for peripheral DE proposed by the author (Prasad) is demonstrated in Table 5.7. As noted earlier, BTK CTOs are often calcified and may contain thrombus. Tips to avoid DE include use of aggressive vasodilators, limiting orbital or rotational atherectomy run times, and maintaining adequate antithrombin and antiplatelet therapy. EPDs, including filters, may be helpful at preventing macrovascular DE and should be considered when the target vessel is appropriately sized. Use of distal filters with orbital or specific rotational devices is considered off-label, and an understanding of device-filter compatibility should be made prior to use. In our practice, we have found it rarely necessary to use EPDs (Nav-6, Abbott Vascular) with orbital atherectomy. Rather we follow the tips noted above. Given the availability of small size (3–4 mm) Spider (Medtronic) filters, we often couple directional atherectomy with EPDs when vessel size will allow. Spasm around the filter site can occur, but generally responds to intra-arterial nitroglycerin. Appropriate sizing of the filter to 1.5× vessel diameter is helpful. Material within the filter can embolize during retrieval, and we recommend a partial capture. This technique entails closure of the filter aperture with the retrieval catheter but not complete internalization of the filter – and potentially avoids "cheese grating" of material through the pores. Lastly, EPDs can add significant cost to a case ($500–$1000), and there are a lack of randomized data. Decisions regarding use of these devices should be made on a case by case basis (Table 5.7).

5.7.2   Perforation

Perforation is a serious complication which any CLI operator working in the tibial region must be willing to recognize and treat immediately. The location of perforation within the tibial anatomy has important implications. Due to their location in the calf, proximal tibial perforations are more serious and are likely to increase the risk of compartment syndrome. The anterior compartment tends to be less forgiving, and bleeding into this space is more likely to result in symptoms. In addition, given the depth of the vessel, perforation of the peroneal artery has to be addressed more promptly regardless of the location along the vessel. There are several options to manage extravasation once a perforation is recognized. First inflation of an external blood pressure cuff to two thirds of systemic pressure around the calf can be performed. The cuff inflation should be maintained for 3–5 min intervals.

Table 5.7 Proposed classification of distal embolism events

Distal embolization type	Manifestation	Comments
Type I	Subclinical – embolic high-intensity signals (HITS) detected by ultrasound	Unknown significance; commonly occurs during most endovascular procedures
Type II	Subclinical – small distal vessel cutoffs or loss of microvascular blush	Has little immediate clinical impact but longer-term relevance is unknown
Type III	Clinical – slow flow in macro-vessels without visible thrombus	Can be seen after atherectomy. Often responds to vasodilators (calcium channel blockers or adenosine)
Type IV	Clinical – slow or no flow in macro-vessels with visible embolus	Macro-embolism can be related to thrombus or atherosclerotic debris Can respond to aspiration thrombectomy, use of intravascular glycoprotein 2b/3a inhibitors, or thrombolysis
Type V	Clinical – no flow in major vessel without visible embolus	May occur due to extensive microvascular congestion from diffuse embolization. May respond to vasodilators or thrombolysis. Intravascular ultrasound may be helpful to differentiate dissection from no-reflow

Second, inflation of an intravascular balloon to low atmospheric pressure to prevent continued inflow should be considered. Again intervals should last anywhere between 3 and 5 min. The third option should be reserved for large perforations and includes reversal of anticoagulation with protamine and consideration of more aggressive endovascular therapies. Options include use of a covered stents and branch or even main vessel coiling. Involving a surgeon for continued bleeding is important as the concern for compartment syndrome is high in refractory cases.

5.8   Conclusions

For the majority of patients presenting with CLI, revascularization of BTK CTOs remains the focus of successful limb salvage. Over the past decade, advances in technology and techniques have allowed vascular specialists to treat more complex disease including calcified and long occluded vessels. A careful approach to procedural planning including comfort with retrograde approaches and complication management is central to successful BTK CTO therapy.

References

1. Mendes JJ, Neves J. Diabetic foot infections: current diagnosis and treatment. J Diabet Foot Complications. 2012;4:26–45.
2. Rosfors S, Kanni L, Nystrom T. The impact of transcutaneous oxygen pressure measurements in patients with suspected critical lower limb ischemia. Int Angiol. 2016;35(5):492–7.
3. Manzi M, Cester G, Palena LM, Alek J, Candeo A, Ferraresi R. Vascular imaging of the foot: the first step toward endovascular recanalization. Radiographics Rev Publ Radiol Soc N Am Inc. 2011;31:1623–36.
4. Faglia E, Clerici G, Caminiti M, Curci V, Clerissi J, Losa S, Casini A, Morabito A. Mortality after major amputation in diabetic patients with critical limb ischemia who did and did not undergo previous peripheral revascularization Data of a cohort study of 564 consecutive diabetic patients. J Diabetes Complicat. 2010;24:265–9.
5. Faglia E, Clerici G, Clerissi J, Gabrielli L, Losa S, Mantero M, Caminiti M, Curci V, Quarantiello A, Lupattelli T, Morabito A. Long-term prognosis of diabetic patients with critical limb ischemia: a population-based cohort study. Diabetes Care. 2009;32:822–7.
6. Goodney PP, Travis LL, Nallamothu BK, Holman K, Suckow B, Henke PK, Lucas FL, Goodman DC, Birkmeyer JD, Fisher ES. Variation in the use of lower extremity vascular procedures for critical limb ischemia. Circ Cardiovasc Qual Outcomes. 2012;5:94–102.
7. Gray BH, Diaz-Sandoval LJ, Dieter RS, Jaff MR, White CJ. Peripheral Vascular Disease Committee for the Society for Cardiovascular A and Interventions. SCAI expert consensus statement for infrapopliteal arterial intervention appropriate use. Catheter Cardiovasc Interv Off J Soc Cardiac Angiography Interv. 2014;84:539–45.
8. Norgren L, Hiatt WR, Dormandy JA, Nehler MR, Harris KA, Fowkes FG, Group TIW. Inter-society consensus for the management of peripheral arterial disease (TASC II). J Vasc Surg. 2007;45 Suppl S:S5–67.
9. Norgren L, Hiatt WR, Harris KA, Lammer J, Group TIW. TASC II section F on revascularization in PAD. J Endovasc Ther Off J Int Soc Endovasc Spec. 2007;14:743–4.

10. Lyden SP, Smouse HB. TASC II and the endovascular management of infrainguinal disease. J Endovasc Ther Off J Int Soc Endovasc Spec. 2009;16:II5–18.
11. Romiti M, Albers M, Brochado-Neto FC, Durazzo AE, Pereira CA, De Luccia N. Meta-analysis of infrapopliteal angioplasty for chronic critical limb ischemia. J Vasc Surg. 2008;47:975–81.
12. Adam DJ, Beard JD, Cleveland T, Bell J, Bradbury AW, Forbes JF, Fowkes FG, Gillepsie I, Ruckley CV, Raab G, Storkey H, BASIL trial participants. Bypass versus angioplasty in severe ischaemia of the leg (BASIL): multicentre, randomised controlled trial. Lancet. 2005;366:1925–34.
13. Rocha-Singh KJ, Jaff M, Joye J, Laird J, Ansel G, Schneider P, VIVA Physicians. Major adverse limb events and wound healing following infrapopliteal artery stent implantation in patients with critical limb ischemia: the XCELL trial. Catheter Cardiovasc Interv Off J Soc Cardiac Angiography Interv. 2012;80:1042–51.
14. Katib N, Thomas SD, Lennox AF, Yang JL, Varcoe RL. An Endovascular-First Approach to the Treatment of Critical Limb Ischemia Results in Superior Limb Salvage Rates. J Endovasc Ther Off J Int Soc Endovasc Spec. 2015;22:473–81.
15. Bradbury AW, Adam DJ, Bell J, Forbes JF, Fowkes FG, Gillespie I, Ruckley CV, Raab GM, Participants B. Bypass versus Angioplasty in Severe Ischaemia of the Leg (BASIL) trial: analysis of amputation free and overall survival by treatment received. J Vasc Surg. 2010;51:18S–31S.
16. Bradbury AW, Adam DJ, Bell J, Forbes JF, Fowkes FG, Gillespie I, Ruckley CV, Raab GM, Participants B. Bypass versus Angioplasty in Severe Ischaemia of the Leg (BASIL) trial: an intention-to-treat analysis of amputation-free and overall survival in patients randomized to a bypass surgery-first or a balloon angioplasty-first revascularization strategy. J Vasc Surg. 2010;51:5S–17S.
17. Menard MT, Farber A. The BEST-CLI trial: a multidisciplinary effort to assess whether surgical or endovascular therapy is better for patients with critical limb ischemia. Semin Vasc Surg. 2014;27:82–4.
18. McCoach CE, Armstrong EJ, Singh S, Javed U, Anderson D, Yeo KK, Westin GG, Hedayati N, Amsterdam EA, Laird JR. Gender-related variation in the clinical presentation and outcomes of critical limb ischemia. Vasc Med. 2013;18:19–26.
19. Iida O, Soga Y, Yamauchi Y, Hirano K, Kawasaki D, Tazaki J, Yamaoka T, Suematsu N, Suzuki K, Shintani Y, Miyashita Y, Takahara M, Uematsu M. Anatomical predictors of major adverse limb events after infrapopliteal angioplasty for patients with critical limb ischaemia due to pure isolated infrapopliteal lesions. Eur J Vasc Endovasc Surg J Off J Eur Soc Vasc Surg. 2012;44:318–24.
20. Alexandrescu V, Hubermont G. Primary infragenicular angioplasty for diabetic neuroischemic foot ulcers following the angiosome distribution: a new paradigm for the vascular interventionist? Diabetes Metab Syndr Obes Targets Ther. 2011;4:327–36.
21. Iida O, Nanto S, Uematsu M, Ikeoka K, Okamoto S, Dohi T, Fujita M, Terashi H, Nagata S. Importance of the angiosome concept for endovascular therapy in patients with critical limb ischemia. Catheter Cardiovasc Interv Off J Soc Cardiac Angiography Interv. 2010;75:830–6.
22. Munce NR, Yang VX, Standish BA, Qiang B, Butany J, Courtney BK, Graham JJ, Dick AJ, Strauss BH, Wright GA, Vitkin IA. Ex vivo imaging of chronic total occlusions using forward-looking optical coherence tomography. Lasers Surg Med. 2007;39:28–35.
23. Ruzsa Z, Nemes B, Bansaghi Z, Toth K, Kuti F, Kudrnova S, Berta B, Huttl K, Merkely B. Transpedal access after failed anterograde recanalization of complex below-the-knee and femoropoliteal occlusions in critical limb ischemia. Catheter Cardiovasc Interv Off J Soc Cardiac Angiography Interv. 2014;83:997–1007.
24. Mustapha JA, Saab F, McGoff T, Heaney C, Diaz-Sandoval L, Sevensma M, Karenko B. Tibio-pedal arterial minimally invasive retrograde revascularization in patients with advanced peripheral vascular disease: the TAMI technique, original case series. Catheter Cardiovasc Interv Off J Soc Cardiac Angiography Interv. 2014;83:987–94.

25. Palena LM, Manzi M. Extreme below-the-knee interventions: retrograde transmetatarsal or transplantar arch access for foot salvage in challenging cases of critical limb ischemia. J Endovasc Ther Off J Int Soc Endovasc Spec. 2012;19:805–11.
26. Palena LM, Brocco E, Manzi M. The clinical utility of below-the-ankle angioplasty using "transmetatarsal artery access" in complex cases of CLI. Catheter Cardiovasc Interv Off J Soc Cardiac Angiography Interv. 2014;83:123–9.
27. Lorenzoni R, Roffi M. Transradial access for peripheral and cerebrovascular interventions. J Invasive Cardiol. 2013;25:529–36.
28. Brilakis ES, Grantham JA, Rinfret S, Wyman RM, Burke MN, Karmpaliotis D, Lembo N, Pershad A, Kandzari DE, Buller CE, DeMartini T, Lombardi WL, Thompson CA. A percutaneous treatment algorithm for crossing coronary chronic total occlusions. JACC Cardiovasc Interv. 2012;5:367–79.
29. Banerjee S, Sarode K, Patel A, Mohammad A, Parikh R, Armstrong EJ, Tsai S, Shammas NW, Brilakis ES. Comparative assessment of guidewire and microcatheter vs a crossing device-based strategy to traverse infrainguinal peripheral artery chronic total occlusions. J Endovasc Ther Off J Int Soc Endovasc Spec. 2015;22:525–34.
30. Spinosa DJ, Leung DA, Harthun NL, Cage DL, Fritz Angle J, Hagspiel KD, Matsumoto AH. Simultaneous antegrade and retrograde access for subintimal recanalization of peripheral arterial occlusion. J Vasc Interv Radiol JVIR. 2003;14:1449–54.
31. Mustapha JA, Saab F, Diaz L, Karenko B, Richards L, Laeder T, Heaney CM, Das T. Utility and feasibility of ultrasound-guided access in patients with critical limb ischemia. Catheter Cardiovasc Interv Off J Soc Cardiac Angiography Interv. 2013;81:1204–11.
32. Mustapha JA, Diaz-Sandoval LJ. Balloon angioplasty in tibioperoneal interventions for patients with critical limb ischemia. Tech Vasc Interv Radiol. 2014;17:183–96.
33. Sarode K, Spelber DA, Bhatt DL, Mohammad A, Prasad A, Brilakis ES, Banerjee S. Drug delivering technology for endovascular management of infrainguinal peripheral artery disease. JACC Cardiovasc Interv. 2014;7:827–39.
34. Trombert D, Caradu C, Brizzi V, Berard X, Midy D, Ducasse E. Evidence for the use of drug eluting stents in below-the-knee lesions. J Cardiovasc Surg. 2015;56:67–71.
35. Liistro F, Porto I, Angioli P, Grotti S, Ricci L, Ducci K, Falsini G, Ventoruzzo G, Turini F, Bellandi G, Bolognese L. Drug-eluting balloon in peripheral intervention for below the knee angioplasty evaluation (DEBATE-BTK): a randomized trial in diabetic patients with critical limb ischemia. Circulation. 2013;128:615–21.
36. Zeller T, Baumgartner I, Scheinert D, Brodmann M, Bosiers M, Micari A, Peeters P, Vermassen F, Landini M, Snead DB, Kent KC, Rocha-Singh KJ, Investigators IPDT. Drug-eluting balloon versus standard balloon angioplasty for infrapopliteal arterial revascularization in critical limb ischemia: 12-month results from the IN.PACT DEEP randomized trial. J Am Coll Cardiol. 2014;64:1568–76.
37. Bhatt P, Parikh P, Patel A, Chag M, Chandarana A, Parikh R, Parikh K. Orbital atherectomy system in treating calcified coronary lesions: 3-year follow-up in first human use study (ORBIT I trial). Cardiovasc Revasc Med Incl Mol Interv. 2014;15:204–8.
38. Staniloae CS, Korabathina R. Orbital atherectomy: device evolution and clinical data. J Invasive Cardiol. 2014;26:215–9.
39. Zeller T, Krankenberg H, Steinkamp H, Rastan A, Sixt S, Schmidt A, Sievert H, Minar E, Bosiers M, Peeters P, Balzer JO, Gray W, Tubler T, Wissgott C, Schwarzwalder U, Scheinert D. One-year outcome of percutaneous rotational atherectomy with aspiration in infrainguinal peripheral arterial occlusive disease: the multicenter pathway PVD trial. J Endovasc Ther Off J Int Soc Endovasc Spec. 2009;16:653–62.
40. Laird JR, Zeller T, Gray BH, Scheinert D, Vranic M, Reiser C, Biamino G, Investigators L. Limb salvage following laser-assisted angioplasty for critical limb ischemia: results of the LACI multicenter trial. J Endovasc Ther Off J Int Soc Endovasc Spec. 2006;13:1–11.
41. Henry M, Amor M, Ethevenot G, Henry I, Allaoui M. Percutaneous peripheral atherectomy using the rotablator: a single-center experience. J Endovasc Surg Off J Int Soc Endovasc Surg. 1995;2:51–66.

42. McKinsey JF, Zeller T, Rocha-Singh KJ, Jaff MR, Garcia LA, DEFINITIVE LE Investigators. Lower extremity revascularization using directional atherectomy: 12-month prospective results of the DEFINITIVE LE study. JACC Cardiovasc Interv. 2014;7:923–33.

43. Shammas NW, Shammas GA, Dippel EJ, Jerin M, Shammas WJ. Predictors of distal embolization in peripheral percutaneous interventions: a report from a large peripheral vascular registry. J Invasive Cardiol. 2009;21:628–31.

44. Reeves R, Imsais JK, Prasad A. Successful management of lower extremity distal embolization following percutaneous atherectomy with the JetStream G3 device. J Invasive Cardiol. 2012;24:E124–8.

45. Zafar N, Prasad A, Mahmud E. Utilization of an aspiration thrombectomy catheter (Pronto) to treat acute atherothrombotic embolization during percutaneous revascularization of the lower extremity. Catheter Cardiovasc Interv Off J Soc Cardiac Angiography Interv. 2008;71:972–5.

46. Shammas NW, Dippel EJ, Shammas G, Gayton L, Coiner D, Jerin M. Dethrombosis of the lower extremity arteries using the power-pulse spray technique in patients with recent onset thrombotic occlusions: results of the DETHROMBOSIS Registry. J Endovasc Ther Off J Int Soc Endovasc Spec. 2008;15:570–9.

47. Keo H, Diehm N, Baumgartner R, Husmann M, Baumgartner I. Single center experience with provisional abciximab therapy in complex lower limb interventions. VASA Zeitschrift fur Gefasskrankheiten. 2008;37:257–64.

48. Manzi M, Palena LM. Treating calf and pedal vessel disease: the extremes of intervention. Semin Intervent Radiol. 2014;31(4):313–9.

Chapter 6
Comparative Assessment of Crossing and Reentry Devices in Treating Chronic Total Occlusions for Femoropopliteal and Below-the-Knee Interventions

Nicolas W. Shammas

Chronic total occlusions (CTOs) are widely prevalent in peripheral arterial interventions. It is estimated that CTOs are encountered in 25–50% of all lesions treated [1]. Multiple predictors of failure to cross CTO have been reported including lesion length, the presence of side branches at the proximal or distal cap, heavily calcified vessels, and operator's experience. A failure rate of up to 50% has been reported when intraluminal crossing of a CTO was attempted with conventional guidewires [2, 3] but significantly improved with specialized crossing devices into the 70% range [3]. A subintimal approach is likely to have a higher initial success rate in the 80% range, but this is dependent on operator's familiarity with reentry devices and lack of severe calcification at the reentry site. Also a higher loss of patency is seen with an initial subintimal approach on intermediate-term follow-up [4–6]. In all comers, the overall technical failure rate remains high at approximately 20% with conventional guidewires and balloons [2, 7]. In this chapter we review published data on CTO devices in peripheral interventions. Randomized comparisons of the effectiveness and safety of these devices in treating CTO are lacking. We therefore present observational studies and non-randomized comparisons between these devices while acknowledging the significant limitations of the data.

Recent advances in crossing CTO have allowed endovascular specialists to treat these lesions percutaneously rather than by primary surgical bypass. National trends in treating lower extremity peripheral arterial disease indicate that between 2001 and 2007, endovascular interventions increased by 78% and surgical bypasses reduced by 20%. During the same period, total amputations (59,693 vs 50,254, $p < 0.001$), major amputations (39,543 vs 31,043, $p < 0.001$), and minor amputations (20,150 vs 19,211, $p < 0.001$) were all significantly decreased [8]. Percutaneous intervention is

N.W. Shammas, MD, MS, FACC, FSCAI
Midwest Cardiovascular Research Foundation, 1622 E Lombard Street, Davenport, 52803 Iowa, USA

Cardiovascular Medicine, PC, Davenport, Iowa, USA
e-mail: Shammas@mchsi.com

© Springer Science+Business Media Singapore 2017
S. Banerjee (ed.), *Practical Approach to Peripheral Arterial Chronic Total Occlusions*, DOI 10.1007/978-981-10-3053-6_6

likely to be associated with quicker recovery, shorter length of hospital stay, and less acute complications.

Multiple catheters are available for treating CTO. The Crosser® (Bard) and TruePath™ (Boston Scientific) are devices designed for intraluminal crossing. The rotational energy at the tip of the devices is transmitted to the CTO cap where intra-luminal recanalization is achieved in 75% and 80%, respectively [9, 10]. Also, the Cordis Frontrunner™ XP (Cordis Corp.) uses microdissections as it enters the plaque, whereas the Viance™ (Medtronic) relies on a fast spin of its atraumatic tip for crossing. The Wildcat™ (Avinger, Inc.) uses spiral wedges on the tip of the catheter that corkscrew the CTO. Finally, the Ocelot™ (Avinger, Inc.) uses optical coherence tomography (OCT) to visualize the lumen as it crosses the occlusion.

6.1   Definitions

In order to meaningfully compare between devices and strategies, it is important to have standardized definitions to what constitutes technical success and procedural success in treating CTO [3]. Technical success is defined as the placement of a guidewire in the distal true lumen past the distal CTO cap confirmed by either angi-ography or intravascular ultrasound. Technical success can be primary, secondary, or provisional. Primary success is a successful crossing with the initial crossing strategy, whereas secondary success is a failure to cross with the initial strategy but achieving success with the use of an alternate crossing device. Provisional success is subintimal passage with the initial crossing strategy with subsequent successful intraluminal crossing with reentry device. Finally, procedural success is obtaining less than or equal 30% residual narrowing at the end of the treatment of a CTO.

6.2   Primary Crossing Devices Versus Primary Wire-Catheter as Initial Crossing Strategy

Data from the Excellence in Peripheral Arterial Disease (XLPAD) registry [3] have demonstrated that an initial strategy with the use of a crossing device leads to a higher chance of crossing success when compared to the use of guidewires and catheters. Four-hundred and thirty-eight CTO lesions were analyzed from the XLPAD registry. Two-hundred and ninety-five (67.4%) lesions were treated with primary wire-cathe-ter and 143 (32.6%) with primary CTO crossing device. Switching to a CTO crossing device and use of reentry device were more frequent in the wire-catheter versus the crossing device strategy (28.1% vs 4.9% and 26.7% vs 17.5%, respectively). Primary technical success was higher in the CTO device versus wire-catheter strategy (72.1% vs 51.9%, respectively, $p < 0.001$), but secondary technical success (71.4% vs 67.5%, $p = 1.0$), provisional technical success (87.5% vs 84.2%, $p = 0.768$), and procedural success (90.9% vs 93.6%, respectively, $p = 0.332$) were similar between the two groups, respectively. In addition, the use of CTO devices was associated with longer procedural times, more contrast use, and longer fluoroscopy times. Furthermore, 30-day and 1-year outcomes were similar between both groups, but there was a significantly higher surgical revascularization rate in the primary wire-catheter arm (8.8% vs 2.8%, $p = 0.025$). Finally, the improvement in the Rutherford-Becker category and ankle brachial index (ABI) was also similar between the two groups when compared to baseline. Viance™ and Frontrunner™ devices were the predominant crossing devices used in this registry (84%). The Viance™ catheter was mainly used in below-the-knee and popliteal lesions, whereas the Frontrunner™ was used more in the superficial femoral artery lesions (100% vs 64.5%, $p < 0.0001$). This data is limited by its retrospective nature with a likely selection bias to the choice of the crossing device. Also the influence of operator's experience was not taken into account as well as cost-effectiveness of various crossing strategies.

A primary wire strategy followed by a reentry device as bailout has also been shown to be effective in achieving a high technical success in treating a CTO. In a retrospective analysis from Germany, 128 patients with 146 lesions were treated with a wire-only strategy first followed by a reentry strategy in 7 out of 13 lesions that were not successfully crossed. A high technical success was accomplished with a wire-only strategy at 91.9%. When a reentry device was used, technical success was achieved in 100% of cases. The authors concluded that technical success can be achieved in more than 90% of all cases with CTO of the lower extremity using a wire-only strategy, and when a reentry device is used after failure of wire crossing, a technical success rate of 100% can be achieved [11].

It can be concluded that a primary technical success is likely to occur with the initial use of specialized crossing devices instead of conventional guidewires. However, a high secondary technical success is seen when switching to an alternate strategy. This indicates that it may be more cost-effective to use specialized crossing or reentry devices after failure of conventional guidewires. This will likely result in high rates of crossing the CTO and overall procedural success. Table 6.1 summarizes data from several small studies describing technical and procedural success and the use of fluoroscopy and contrast dye with various crossing or reentry devices.

6.3   Crossing Devices (Table 6.1)

6.3.1   TruePath™ (Boston Scientific)

The TruePath™ system (Fig. 6.1) creates microdissection in CTOs to facilitate access into hard and calcified caps. It is a 0.018″ guidewire compatible. The tip (Fig. 6.2) is diamond coated and rotates at 13,000 rpm. It has audible and visual alerts that are activated when excessive resistance is encountered. The tip may be bent up to 15° to help steering it in different directions.

In a small series from the XLPAD registry, 13 patients with mostly TASC C and D lesions and femoropopliteal (FP) CTO were treated with the TruePath™ device after an unsuccessful guidewire crossing attempt. Twelve lesions were de novo and severely calcified. Technical success was 77%. In three patients, subintimal recanalization

Table 6.1 Published literature on intraluminal crossing devices

Devices	n	LL (mm)	De novo (%)	Calcium (%)	Location (%)	TS (%)	Primary TS (%)	Reentry use (%)	PS (%)	Stent (%)	Fluro (min)	Contrast (cc)	References
TruePath	13	169.8	92.3	Severe = 92.3	SFA 77	100	77	23	100 (<30%)	61.5	41	200	[12]
TruePath	85	*	*	Moderate or severe = 85	SFA 71.8	80	*	*	*	*	*	*	[14]
Crosser	73	*	95.9	Moderate or severe = 57.6	*	87.7	76.7	13.7	*	51.6	*	*	[15]
Crosser	85	117.5	*	Moderate or severe = 75	SFA 61.2, pop 20, IP 16.5	83.5	*	*	75.3 (<50%)	51.8	39.1	242	[16]
Viance#	37	81	97	Severe = 41	Pop and IP 100	70	65	4		5	28	189	[39]
Viance	58	140	93.1	Severe = 93.1	SFA 58.6	96.6	87.9	12.1	85.7	51.7	39.1	187	[13]
Frontrunner XP	26	176	*	Heavy = 68	FemPop 100	65.38	*	9	*	*	22.9	*	[17]
Frontrunner XP	22	180	100	Mild = 86.4, Severe = 9.1	FemPop 100	95.5	95.5	*	95.5	*	*	*	[18]
Wildcat	84	174	88.6	Moderate = 57; Severe = 1.2	SFA 85.2	89	75	17.8	89.8 (<50%)	34.1	30.2	247	[19]
Ocelot	100	16.6	89	Moderate = 36	SFA 94, Pop 4, FP 2	97	72	*	97	*	38.6	223	[20]
Ocelot	33	205	94	Severe = 21, Moderate = 12	SFA 100	100	83.9	16	*	71	28	132	[21]

Viance and CrossBoss, * missing info, SFA superficial femoral artery, Pop popliteal, IP infrapopliteal, Fempop femoropopliteal, cc ml, TS technical success, PS procedural success, min minute, Fluro fluoroscopy, LL lesion length, Reentry use reentry device use, n number

Fig. 6.1 TruePath™ system (© 2015 Boston Scientific. Image(s) used with permission)

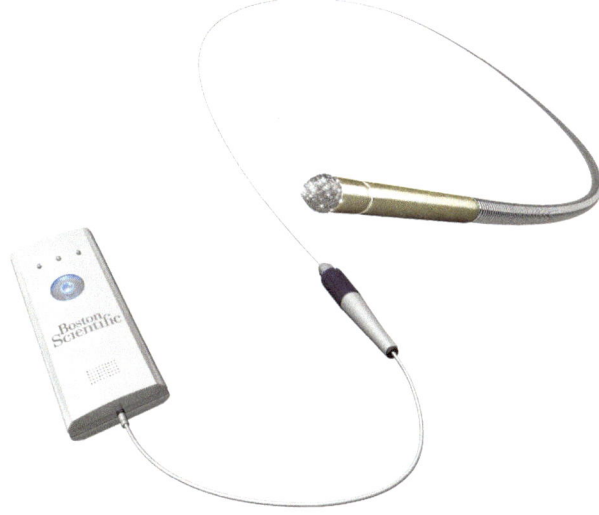

Fig. 6.2 TruePath™ tip is diamond coated and rotates at 13,000 rpm (© 2015 Boston Scientific. Image(s) used with permission)

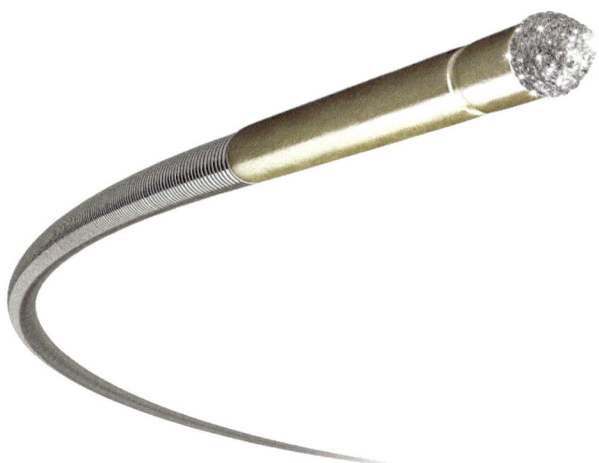

occurred requiring the use of reentry device. Sixty-two percent of patients were stented, and average fluoroscopy time was 41.1 min and contrast use 200 mL [12]. Also Bosiers et al. [14] reported results of the ReOpen trial in which 85 CTO lesions were treated with the TruePath™ device. Moderate or severe calcifications were present in 85% of lesions. Technical success was achieved in 80%. Figure 6.3 illustrates CTO crossed successfully with TruePath™ with establishing intraluminal wire position.

6.3.2   Viance™ (Medtronic)

The Viance™ catheter (Fig. 6.4) has a 2.3 Fr shaft made of coiled multiwire and a 3 Fr rounded atraumatic tip. It is an over the wire and is 0.014″ guidewire compatible. The tip is advanced to the proximal CTO cap and manually spun using a torqueable

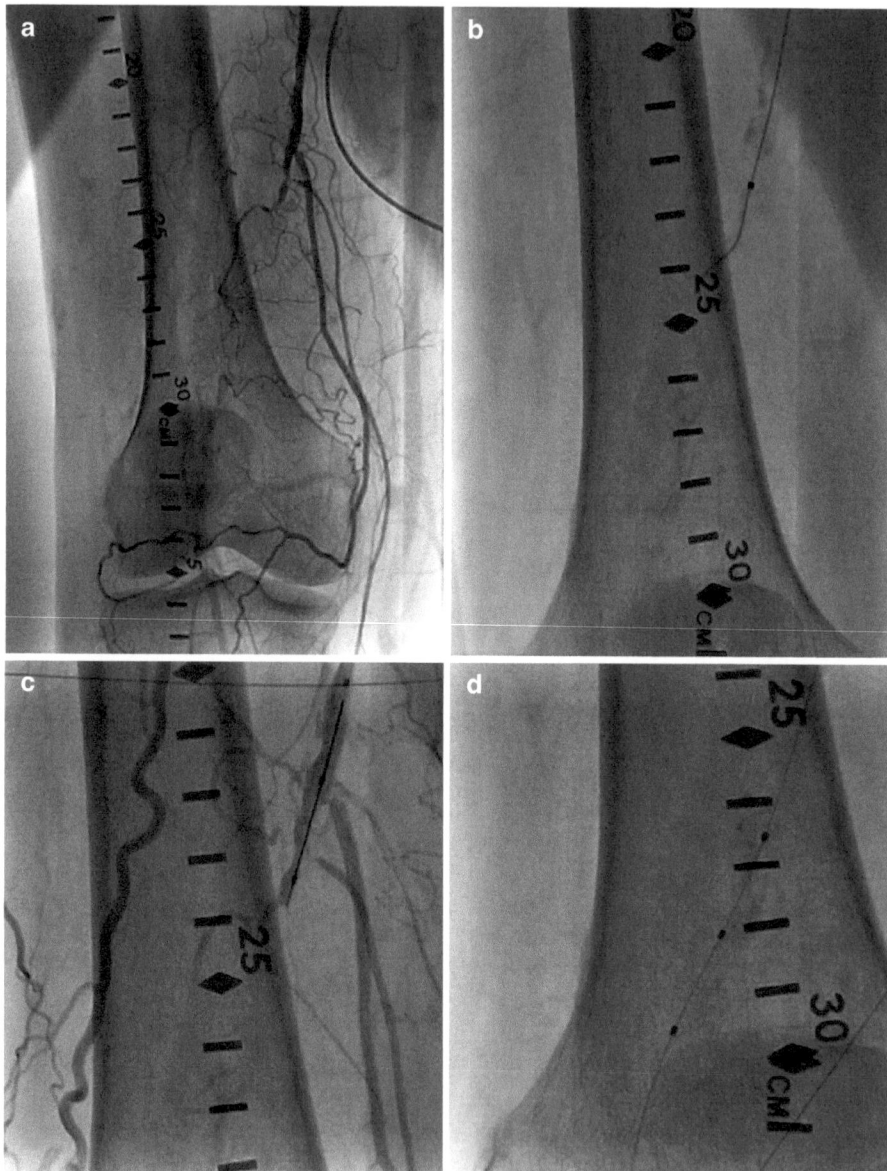

Fig. 6.3 Chronic total occlusion (**a**) could not be crossed with angled-tip extra-stiff glide wire (deflecting into a side branch), (**b**) was engaged successfully with TruePath™ (**c**) (Boston Scientific), and intraluminally successfully crossed (**d**)

handle (Fig. 6.5). Using a "fast spin technique" and forward pushability, the Viance™ tip passes through the CTO via the true lumen or subintimally. The Viance™ has an angulated tip that helps navigating staying away from a side branch at the caps. Also as the device is advanced forward, the wire is retracted proximal to the tip.

Fig. 6.4 Viance™ catheter (© 2015 Medtronic. Image(s) used with permission)

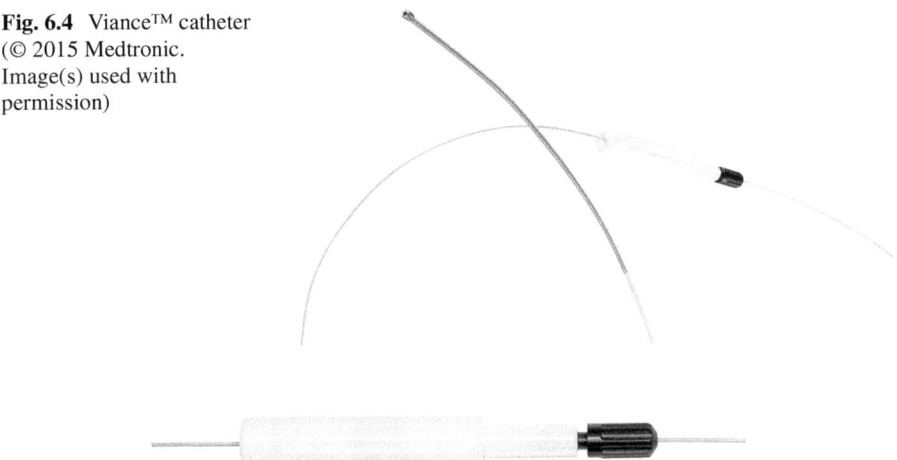

Fig. 6.5 Viance™ torqueable handle (© 2015 Medtronic. Image(s) used with permission)

Fifty-eight patients from the Excellence in Peripheral Artery Disease (XLPAD) registry were treated with the Viance™ catheter; mean lesion length was 140.0 mm; 93.1% of lesions were de novo, and 81.0% were severely calcified [12]. Primary technical success was 87.9% of cases, and procedural success was 85.7%. It should be noted that the technical success was significantly less with the Viance™ after an unsuccessful attempt by the guidewire (50%) when compared to 95.8% after an initial Viance™ crossing attempt. The Viance™ entered the subintimal space in 12.1% of cases, and a reentry device was used. Reentry device success was 71.4%. Additional data from the same registry with application exclusively to below-the-knee CTO achieved primary technical success in 65% of lesions treated. In this registry, 37 lesions were treated with the Viance™ or the CrossBoss™ catheters; mean lesion length was 81 mm, and 41% of lesions are severely calcified. Subintimal entry was achieved in 14% of lesions. Procedural success was achieved in 85.7% of lesions successfully crossed. The main predictor of procedural failure was long lesion length with mean length of 136 mm.

6.3.3   Frontrunner™ XP (FR-XP) (Cordis)

The FR-XP catheter has no guidewire lumen. It consists of a proximal braided shaft to assist in pushability and torque and a flexible distal shaft that can be manually shaped. The radiopaque distal actuating tip is made of a set of bilateral hinged pieces. The device creates a blunt microdissection through a CTO which enables intraluminal guidewire entry. A micro-guide catheter is recommended for use with the FR-XP to provide additional support to the distal portion of the crossing device and also to facilitate guidewire placement into the CTO. The FR-XP is placed through the

Fig. 6.6 Frontrunner™
creating a larger
microdissection plane into
the chronic total occlusion
(©2015 Cordis, Image(s)
used with permission)

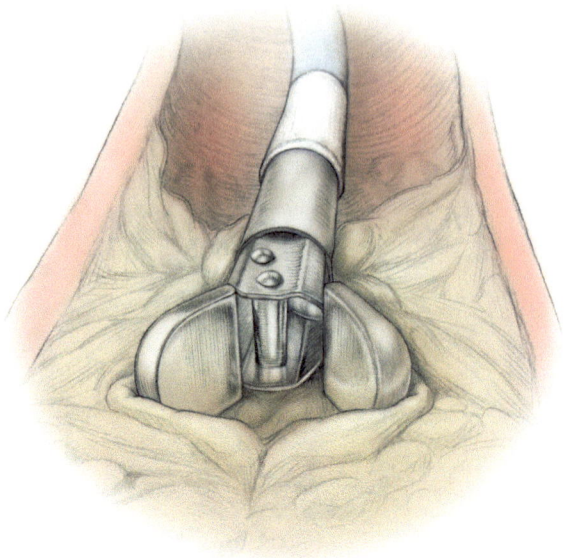

proximal cap of the CTO with jaws closed and then repeatedly pulled back with an "open jaw." This allows a larger microdissection plane into the CTO (Fig. 6.6).

Charalambous et al. [17] treated 26 SFA CTO with the Frontrunner™ catheter following failure of conventional guidewire crossing. Severe calcification was present in 68% of the lesions, and the mean lesion length was 17.6 cm. Technical success was 65.4%. Predictors of failure were severe calcification and inability to reenter the lumen after successful subintimal passage [13, 17]. The mean fluoroscopy time was 22.9 min. Also Shetty et al. [18] treated 22 patients with femoropopliteal CTO (mean occlusion length, 18.0 ± 10.1 cm) with the Frontrunner™ XP catheter after guidewire failure. Technical success was 95.5%.

6.4   Crosser® Catheter System (Bard)

The Crosser® CTO Recanalization System is comprised of an electronic generator, foot switch, high-frequency transducer, the FlowMate® Injector, and Crosser® catheter. It is both 0.014″ and 0.018″ guidewire compatible. The tip is metal (either stainless steel or titanium) and uses high energy vibration to penetrate hard caps. The guidewire is advanced to the site of the occlusion. The Crosser® catheter (Fig. 6.7) is then passed over the guidewire until it reaches the occlusion (Fig. 6.7a). Following pulling back the guidewire, the device is activated and slowly advanced into the lesion.

Staniloae et al. [15] reported on 56 subjects with 73 CTOs who were treated with the Crosser® device. Primary technical success was 76.7%. Secondary technical success was 87.7%. A higher technical success was seen in CTOs in the aortoiliac (90.0%) and tibial (95.2%) vessels. The mean time to cross the CTO was 17.6 min.

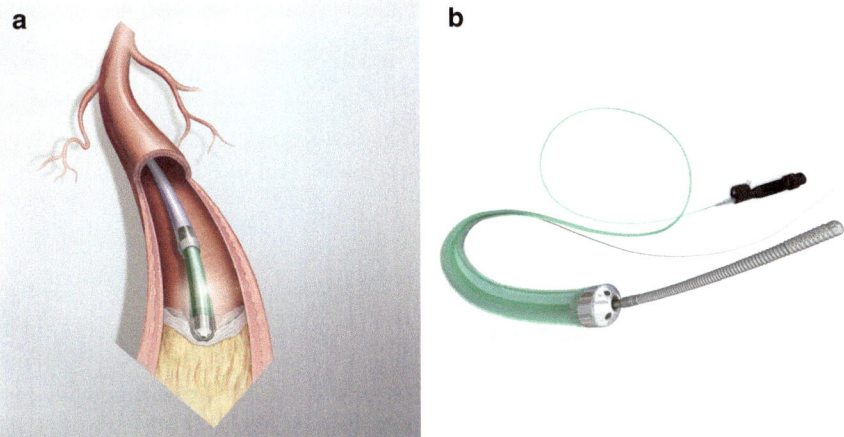

Fig. 6.7 (**a**) Crosser® CTO catheter (© 2015 C. R. Bard, Inc. Image(s) used with permission). (**b**) Crosser® CTO catheter engaging total occlusion (© 2015 C. R. Bard, Inc. Image(s) used with permission)

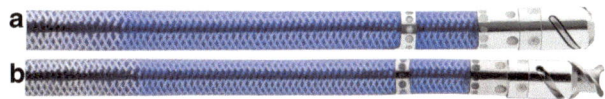

Fig. 6.8 Wildcat™ with a rotatable tip that can assume both passive (wedges in, **a**) and active (wedges out, **b**) configurations (© 2015 Avinger, Inc. Image(s) used with permission)

No perforations were reported. Longer lesions (>100 mm) and calcification within 10 mm of the exit cap were predictors of failure to cross. More recently, Laird et al. [16] reported the results of the PATRIOT trial. In this study, 85 patients with failure to cross a CTO with conventional guidewires were treated with the Crosser® device. Vessels treated included the superficial femoral artery in 61.2%, popliteal artery 20%, and tibioperoneal arteries in 16.5%. Mean occlusion length was 117.5 mm with 75% were moderately to severely calcified. Technical success was 83.5% with zero Crosser® catheter-related perforations. Procedural success was 75.3% (≤50% residual stenosis). Average Crosser® catheter activation time was 2 min and 6 s.

6.4.1   Wildcat™ (Avinger)

The Wildcat™ has a rotatable tip that can assume both passive (wedges in) and active (wedges out) configurations (Fig. 6.8a, b). The passive mode is the recommended initial mode. For fibrocalcific lesions, the active mode is used. Recently, a handheld motorized unit can be used to rotate the device. The 0.014″ versions of this device (Kittycat and Kittycat 2) may allow better crossability of smaller vessels for both above-the-knee or tibial lesions.

In a multicenter study at 15 US sites, 84 patients with CTO were treated with the Wildcat™ crossing catheter per protocol after an initial failure attempt using conventional guidewires. Technical success was 89% ($n = 75$). Primary technical success was 75%. Five percent of cases had major adverse events (minor perforations sealed with balloon angioplasty). Of the 75 patients successfully crossed, 17.8% required the use of a reentry device which was successful in 80%. Procedural success was 89.8% [19].

6.4.2 Ocelot™ (Avinger)

The Ocelot™ CTO crossing device (Fig. 6.9a) is an over-the-wire device with optical coherence tomography (OCT) imaging capability and consists of a catheter shaft with crossing distal tip and a proximal handle assembly. OCT's infrared spectrum is reliable in identifying plaque morphology [22, 23] and provides continuous A-scans that are translated into extrapolated images that guide navigating the tip within the CTO. The OCT image generated by the Ocelot™ catheter is related to the device's orientation (Fig. 6.9b). The distal tip of the catheter consists of spiral flutes and a fiber optic used in conjunction with a light box to help in directing the intravascular tip position using directional markers. The latter remains stationary in the OCT display unless the outer shaft of the catheter is rotated. The device is not intended for use in the coronary, iliac, renal, carotid, or cerebral vessels.

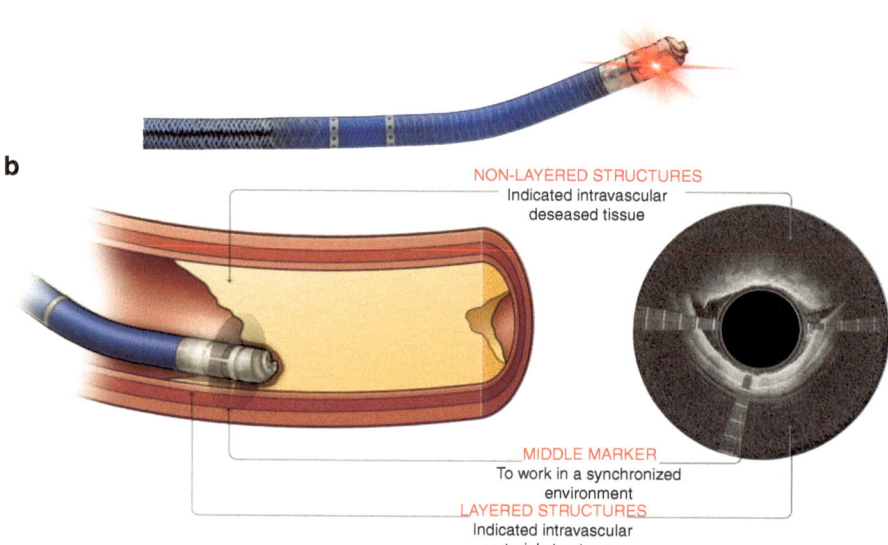

a

b

NON-LAYERED STRUCTURES
Indicated intravascular
deseased tissue

MIDDLE MARKER
To work in a synchronized
environment
LAYERED STRUCTURES
Indicated intravascular
arterial structures

Fig. 6.9 (**a**) Ocelot™ CTO crossing device (© 2015 Avinger, Inc. Image(s) used with permission). (**b**) The OCT image generated by the Ocelot™ catheter is related to the device's orientation (© 2015 Avinger, Inc. Image(s) used with permission)

In the CONNECT II study, a prospective, multicenter, nonrandomized single-arm study evaluating the safety and effectiveness of the Ocelot™ catheter in CTO crossing that could not be crossed with a guidewire, 100 patients (94% superficial femoral artery, mean lesion length 16.6 mm) were included. The primary technical success was 72%, and the overall technical success was 97%. A reentry device was used in 7% of patients [20]. Also Schwindt et al. [21] reported their data on 33 patients with SFA CTO crossed with the Ocelot™ catheter. Technical success was 100% despite mean lesion length of 205 mm. Primary technical success was 83.9%. Reentry device was used in 16% of cases, and stent rate was 71%.

When the Ocelot™ was compared to the Wildcat™ using data from CONNECT [19], a significant reduction in procedure time and contrast use were obtained with the OCT-guided Ocelot™ catheter. There was, however, no significant difference in the rate of perforations, embolizations, or dissections. Although numerically the Ocelot™ had a better ability to cross the CTO than the Wildcat™ (100% vs 95.2%), this was not statistically significant. When a select cohort of Ocelot™ patients who met the inclusion and exclusion criteria of the CONNECT study were separately analyzed, the CTO was successfully crossed in 100% of the time.

6.5   Reentry Devices (Table 6.2)

6.5.1   Subintimal Angioplasty of CTO Lesions

Subintimal angioplasty (SIA) is an effective, low-cost, and easy-to-learn method in treating femoropopliteal CTO. The immediate- and short-term results are encouraging. In addition to improving claudication, limb salvage has been demonstrated in

Table 6.2 Published literature on reentry devices

Devices	n	LL (mm)	De novo (%)	Location (%)	TS (%)	Procedural success (%)	Stent (%)	Fluro (min)	References
Outback LTD	52	176	100	SFA 90.4, SFA/pop 9.6	64.5	*	*	*	[24]
Outback	51	230	100	Iliac15.7, FP 82.3	96.1	96.1	96.1	*	[25]
Outback	65	200	100	SFA 100	88	88	*	*	[26]
Outback	26	*	100	*	100	*	*	29.8	[27]
Pioneer	25	127	100	SFA 100	100	100 (<25%)	100	*	[28]
Pioneer	21	iliacs 8.5, SFA 1.5	100	Iliac 18, SFA 3	100	*	100	38	[1]
OffRoad	92	175.1	100	SFA/Pop	84.8	*	*	21	[29]
Enteer	21	*	*	*	86	*	*	*	Unpublished#

n number, *LL* lesion length, *mm* millimeter, *TS* technical success, *Fluro* fluoroscopy, *min* minute, *SFA* superficial femoral artery, *Pop* popliteal, *FP* femoropopliteal, # from Boston Sci. web page, * data not available

limb ischemia patient. Unfortunately, SIA is associated with a low patency rate at 1 year ranging from 45% to 62% [30–33]. Predictors of loss of patency in SIA include long lesions, limb ischemia, and diabetics. Furthermore, a subintimal approach is associated with a high rate of dissection and stenting. Finally, a subintimal approach nearly eliminates the possibility of atherectomy as a first-line treatment. Although some reports indicated that SIA may reduce distal embolization [34], this has not been demonstrated consistently in all studies [35, 36]. This approach, in our laboratory, is limited only to patients in whom an intraluminal approach is demonstrated to be difficult to accomplish successfully. The main reason for SIA failure is reentry into the true lumen, generally hindered by severe calcification at the reentry site or lack of experience of the operator with the device being used. Below is a list of reentry devices that are currently available.

6.5.2 *Pioneer™ (Medtronic)*

The Pioneer™ catheter is 0.014″ wire compatible catheter with a solid-state intravascular ultrasound (IVUS) transducer (Volcano Therapeutics) and a hypo-tube through the lumen with a curved retractable nitinol needle (Fig. 6.10). After subintimal entry and reaching the desired true lumen entry point, the catheter is rotated so the true lumen is at 12 o'clock on the IVUS image. The curved needle tip is then advanced

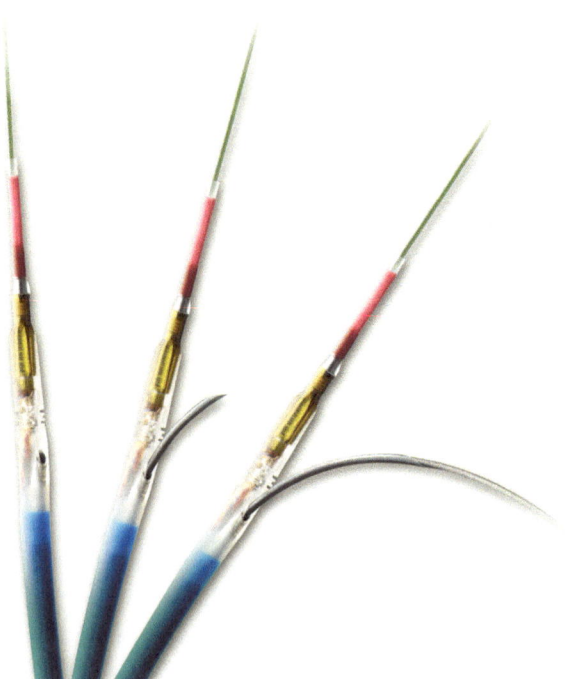

Fig. 6.10 Pioneer™ catheter with a curved retractable nitinol needle

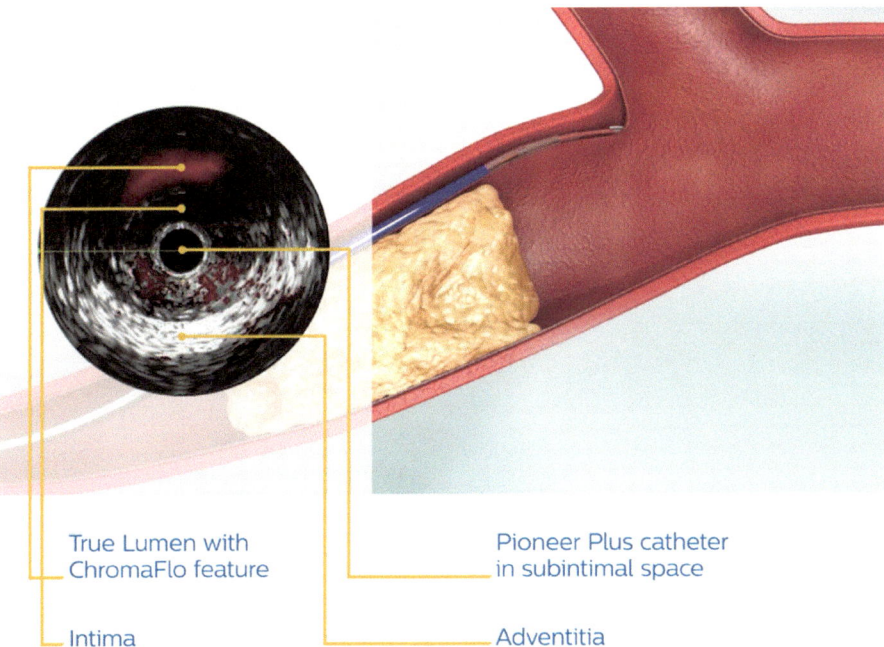

True Lumen with
ChromaFlo feature

Pioneer Plus catheter
in subintimal space

Intima

Adventitia

Fig. 6.11 Pioneer™ retractable needle is retracted and wire crossed intraluminally

away from the IVUS catheter into the true lumen. An exchange length extra-support 0.014″ guidewire is then passed from the needle into the true lumen. The needle is retracted, Pioneer™ catheter withdrawn, and intervention continued (Fig. 6.11).

Jacobs et al. [1] reported on the use of a true lumen reentry device in 24 femoral and iliac CTOs using predominantly the Pioneer™ catheter in 21/24 (87.5%). All 21 vessels treated with the Pioneer™ catheter (18 iliac and 3 SFA) could not be successfully crossed initially by standard catheter, and wire techniques were crossed successfully at a mean of 38 min. No bleeding occurred at the site of true lumen entry. All patients had to be stented. Technical success was 100%. Also, Scheinert et al. [28] reported on 25 consecutive patients with failed attempt to recanalize chronic superficial artery occlusion (mean occlusion length 12.7 cm) with standard techniques and were rescheduled for a secondary recanalization procedure. Technical success was achieved in 100% of cases. Predilatation of the false channel was performed in eight cases with severe calcification to allow advancement of the Pioneer™ catheter. All patients were stented, and procedural success was 100%.

6.5.3 Outback (Cordis)

The Outback catheter (Fig. 6.12) uses a retractable curved nitinol needle positioned under fluoroscopy in two different orthogonal views toward the true lumen. After crossing the subintimal space with a crossing catheter and 0.035″ hydrophilic wire, the 0.035″

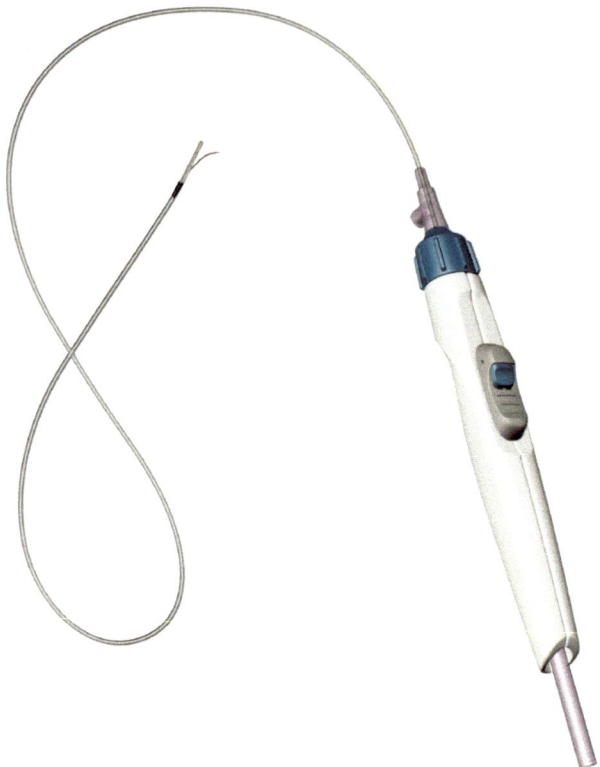

Fig. 6.12 Outback™ catheter (©2015 Cordis. Image(s) used with permission)

wire is then exchanged for a 0.014″ non-hydrophilic support wire (we typically use the Spartacore wire from Abbott). The Outback catheter was then placed over the 0.014″ and advanced under fluoroscopy to the desired reentry site. The L radiopaque marker on the catheter is initially oriented toward the lumen (Fig. 6.13). After rotating the image intensifier 90° orthogonally, the radiopaque marker is simultaneously oriented to form a "T" over the center of the lumen (Fig. 6.13b). The needle is then deployed, guidewire advanced through the needle, and then needle retracted, followed by removal of the Outback catheter while keeping the guidewire into the true lumen (Fig. 6.14).

In a study by Shin et al. [24], 52 lesions were treated with the Outback LTD reentry device (47 SFA and 5 combined SFA/popliteal). Reentry was successful in 64.5% of cases. The main predictor of failure included the presence of moderate or severe calcification at site of reentry. In general failures were related to inability to reenter the lumen (61.1%), acute aortic bifurcation angle (11.1%), device failure (5.6%), and difficulty tracking the device over the wire (16.7%) or the device though the lesion (5.6%). Also Beschorner et al. [26] reported 88% success rate in the recanalization of 65 superficial femoral artery CTOs using the Outback reentry catheter after failure of crossing using conventional guidewires. Lesion length was 200 mm. In addition, Aslam et al. [25] reported a procedural success of 96.1% in crossing 51 CTOs of iliofemoral and femoropopliteal lesions (mean lesion length

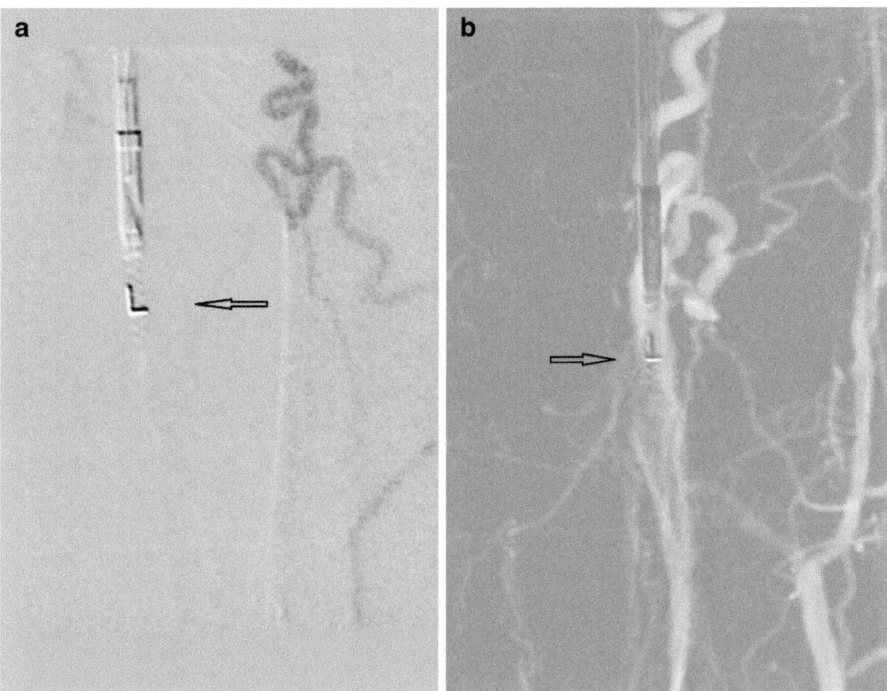

Fig. 6.13 (**a**) The L radiopaque marker on the Outback™ catheter oriented toward the lumen. *Arrow* point to the L marker directed toward lumen (**b**) The radiopaque marker on the Outback catheter™ is simultaneously oriented to form a "T" over the center of the lumen. *Arrow* points to the T marker over the vessel

230 mm) using the Outback LTD catheter. Furthermore, in a small randomized trial by Gandini et al. [27], true lumen reentry was attempted in 52 superficial femoral artery CTO, 26 with conventional guidewires, and 26 with the Outback LTD catheter. Technical success was achieved in 100% of cases. The conventional wire group achieved planned in-target reentry in 42.3%, whereas the Outback group 88.4%. The mean procedural time in the conventional wire group was 55.4 ± 14.2 min with a mean fluoroscopy time 39.6 ± 13.9 min compared to 36.0 ± 9.4 min and 29.8 ± 8.9 min, respectively, in the Outback group. The authors concluded that the use of the Outback reentry was associated with high technical success rates and a significant reduction of procedural and fluoroscopy times.

Recently, Kitrou et al. [37] published their data on 91 patients (100 vessels) with the Outback catheter. All vessels failed initial spontaneous reentry. Fifty-two vessels were iliac occlusion, and 48 were infrainguinal. The Outback was successful in reentry in 93% of cases, and failure to reenter the true lumen was due to severe calcification at the reentry site. There were no major complications reported. A systematic review by the authors on published literature on the Outback catheter noted a successful reentry in 90% of cases with an overall complication rate of 4.3%. The authors concluded that the Outback has a high success rate in reentering the true lumen with low complication rates.

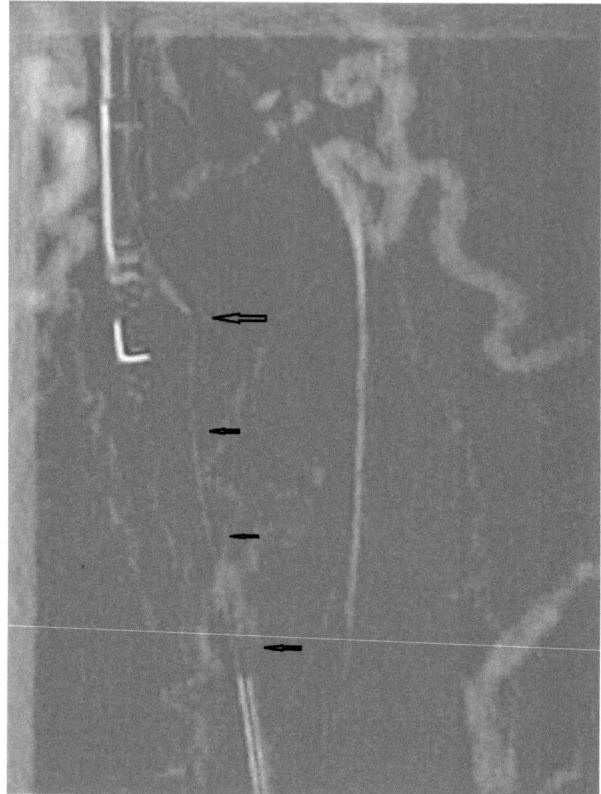

Fig. 6.14 Outback™ catheter removed while keeping the guidewire into the true lumen. *Arrows* point to the wire after crossing into the true lumen

6.5.4 Enteer (Medtronic)

The Enteer Re-entry system (Fig. 6.15) has two components: an orienting balloon catheter and a reentry guidewire. The balloon catheter is indicated for "directing, steering, controlling, and supporting" the guidewire. It has a 150-cm shaft length and is 0.018″ wire compatible. The balloon is flat shape and designed to self-orient one of two 180° offset exit ports toward the true lumen. Enteer can be used for above- and below-the-knee applications. Under fluoroscopic guidance, the balloon is advanced to the planned reentry site. The guidewire is then exchanged with a barbed reentry, angled-tip guidewire with different level of stiffness designed to enter the true lumen from the exit port of the balloon located in the subintimal space. Once true lumen access is accomplished, the reentry balloon is removed, and the barbed wire is exchanged with another guidewire followed by intervention.

In the multicenter (9 US sites) Peripheral Facilitated Antegrade Steering Technique in Chronic Total Occlusions (PFAST) CTO pivotal study, 66 patients with infrainguinal arteries (mean CTO lesion length 19.5 ± 10.8 cm) were included. In 45 cases, the BigBoss (Viance™) was used alone, and in 21 cases, reentry was

Fig. 6.15 Enteer Re-entry system™ (© 2015 Boston Scientific. Image(s) used with permission)

Fig. 6.16 OffRoad Re-entry system™ (© 2015 Boston Scientific. Image(s) used with permission)

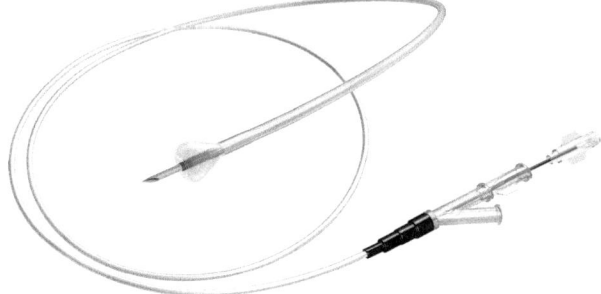

attempted using the Enteer Re-entry system. Overall technical success was 86% (18/21) with the Enteer system. The data of this trial has not been published yet [38].

6.6 OffRoad (Boston Scientific)

The OffRoad Re-entry system (Fig. 6.16) is a dual-component system with a 70 cm over-the-wire 0.035″ compatible catheter system, the tip of which has a 5.4 mm conical-shaped positioning balloon and a flexible neck that allows directing the balloon toward the true lumen and a hollow 0.014″ compatible micro-catheter Lancet with a hydrophilic coating and a lancet tip. The lancet tip is designed to facilitate reentry into the true lumen (Fig. 6.17). The system can be used with a 6 F sheath. After guidewire reaches the desired reentry location, it is removed and replaced by the Lancet micro-catheter. The balloon is then inflated at nominal pressure of two atmospheres (maximum 3.25 ATM) which redirects the balloon toward the true lumen. The Lancet is then advanced into the true lumen followed by advancing the 0.014″ guidewire. The Lancet is retracted and removed, balloon deflated and catheter removed, and intervention continued.

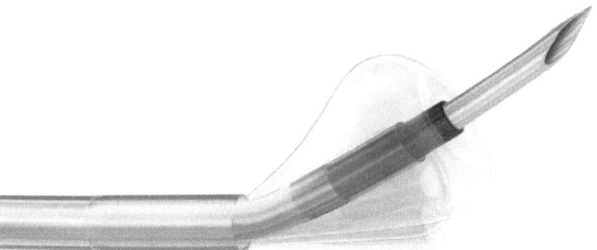

Fig. 6.17 OffRoad™ lancet tip designed to facilitate reentry into the true lumen (© 2015 Boston Scientific. Image(s) used with permission)

Schmidt et al. [29] reported data on the OffRoad Re-entry Catheter System in the femoropopliteal arteries. This single-arm, prospective study of 92 patients with CTO of the femoropopliteal artery was conducted at 12 European centers; technical success was 84.8%. Major adverse events including death, perforation requiring intervention, clinically significant peripheral embolism, and major amputation of the treated lower limb at 30 days were 3.3%.

6.7 Conclusion

Several strategies and devices are now available to the endovascular specialist to treat CTO of infrainguinal arteries. The best strategy is yet to be defined. An initial attempt with a specialized crossing device yields a higher primary technical success than the use of a conventional guidewire; however, after failure of the initial strategy, a second attempt with an alternate strategy seems to yield similar technical success. Provisional technical success with reentry device or a primary subintimal technique is also high, but subintimal intervention carries an overall low patency rate on follow-up, requires a high rate of stenting, and nearly eliminates the use of atherectomy as a primary modality for treatment. Current crossing or reentry devices all enhance technical success. Operator's experience is critical for optimal performance. We recommend that an operator gets familiar with one or two of the crossing and reentry devices and use them frequently enough to build and sustain a high-level experience in crossing CTO.

References

1. Jacobs DL, Motaganahalli RL, Cox DE, Wittgen CM, Peterson GJ. True lumen re-entry devices facilitate subintimal angioplasty and stenting of total chronic occlusions: initial report. J Vasc Surg. 2006;43(6):1291–6.
2. Bolia A, Miles KA, Brennan J, Bell PR. Percutaneous transluminal angioplasty of occlusions of the femoral and popliteal arteries by subintimal dissection. Cardiovasc Interv Radiol. 1990;13:357–63.
3. Banerjee S, Sarode K, Patel A, Mohammad A, Parikh R, Armstrong EJ, Tsai S, Shammas NW, Brilakis ES. Comparative assessment of guidewire and microcatheter vs a crossing device-based strategy to traverse infrainguinal peripheral artery chronic total occlusions. J Endovasc Ther. 2015;22:525–34. pii: 1526602815587707. [Epub ahead of print]

4. London N, Srinivasan R, Naylor A, et al. Subintimal angioplasty of femoropopliteal artery occlusions: the long term results. Eur J Vasc Endovasc Surg. 2011;42(suppl 1):S9–S15.
5. Markose G, Miller FN, Bolia A. Subintimal angioplasty for femoro-popliteal occlusive disease. J Vasc Surg. 2010;52:1410–6.
6. Shammas NW. Subintimal angioplasty and stenting of chronic total femoropopliteal occlusions: is distal protection needed? J Endovasc Ther. 2014;21(4):482–4. doi:10.1583/14-4703C.1.
7. Rogers J, Laird J. Overview of new technologies for lower extremity revascularization. Circulation. 2007;116:2072–85.
8. Hong MS, Beck AW, Nelson PR. Emerging national trends in the management and outcomes of lower extremity peripheral arterial disease. Ann Vasc Surg. 2011;25:44–54.
9. Culverwell AD, Tapping CR, Ettles DF, Kessel D. Patient experience, pain, and quality of life after lower limb angioplasty: a multisite prospective cohort study. Cardiovasc Intervent Radiol. 2012;35:788–94.
10. Gandini R, Volpi T, Pipitone V, Simonetti G. Intraluminal recanalization of long infrainguinal chronic total occlusions using the Crosser System. J Endovasc Ther. 2009;16:23–7.
11. Langhoff R, Stumpe S, Treitl M, Schulte KL. Successful revascularization of chronic total occlusion of lower extremity arteries: a wire only and bail out use of re-entry device approach. J Cardiovasc Surg. 2013;54(5):553–9.
12. Banerjee S, Sarode K, Das T, Hadidi O, Thomas R, Vinas A, Garg P, Mohammad A, Baig MS, Shammas NW, Brilakis ES. Endovascular treatment of infrainguinal chronic total occlusions using the TruePath device: features, handling, and 6-month outcomes. J Endovasc Ther. 2014;21(2):281–8. doi:10.1583/13-4527R.1.
13. Banerjee S, Thomas R, Sarode K, Mohammad A, Sethi S, Baig MS, Gigliotti OS, Ali MI, Klein A, Abu-Fadel MS, Shammas NW, Prasad A, Brilakis ES. Crossing of infrainguinal peripheral arterial chronic total occlusion with a blunt microdissection catheter. J Invasive Cardiol. 2014;26(8):363–9.
14. Bosiers M, Diaz-Cartelle J, Scheinert D, Peeters P, Dawkins KD. Revascularization of lower extremity chronic total occlusions with a novel intraluminal recanalization device: results of the ReOpen study. J Endovasc Ther. 2014;21(1):61–70. doi:10.1583/12-4083R.1.
15. Staniloae CS, Mody KP, Yadav SS, Han SY, Korabathina R. Endoluminal treatment of peripheral chronic total occlusions using the Crosser® recanalization catheter. J Invasive Cardiol. 2011;23(9):359–62.
16. Laird J, Joye J, Sachdev N, Huang P, Caputo R, Mohiuddin I, Runyon J, Das T. Recanalization of infrainguinal chronic total occlusions with the crosser system: results of the PATRIOT trial. J Invasive Cardiol. 2014;26(10):497–504.
17. Charalambous N, Schäfer PJ, Trentmann J, Hümme TH, Stöhring C, Müller-Hülsbeck S, Heller M, Jahnke T. Percutaneous intraluminal recanalization of long, chronic superficial femoral and popliteal occlusions using the Frontrunner XP CTO device: a single-center experience. Cardiovasc Intervent Radiol. 2010;33(1):25–33. doi: 10.1007/s00270-009-9700-x. Epub 2009 Sep 24.
18. Shetty R, Vivek G, Thakkar A, Prasad R, Pai U, Nayak K. Safety and efficacy of the frontrunner XP catheter for recanalization of chronic total occlusion of the femoropopliteal arteries. J Invasive Cardiol. 2013;25(7):344–7.
19. Pigott JP, Raja ML, Davis T; Connect Trial Investigators. A multicenter experience evaluating chronic total occlusion crossing with the Wildcat catheter (the CONNECT study). J Vasc Surg. 2012;56:1615–21. doi: 10.1016/j.jvs.2012.06.071. Epub 2012 Sep 11.
20. Selmon MR, Schwindt AG, Cawich IM, Chamberlin JR, Das TS, Davis TP, George JC, Janzer SF, Lopez LA, McDaniel HB, McKinsey JF, Pigott JP, Raja ML, Reimers B, Schreiber TL. Final results of the chronic total occlusion crossing with the ocelot system II (CONNECT II) study. J Endovasc Ther. 2013;20(6):770–81. doi:10.1583/13-4380MR.1.
21. Schwindt A, Reimers B, Scheinert D, Selmon M, Pigott JP, George JC, Robertson G, Janzer S, McDaniel HB, Shrikhande GV, Torsello G, Schaefers J, Saccà S, Versaci F. Crossing chronic total occlusions with the Ocelot system: the initial European experience. EuroIntervention. 2013;9(7):854–62. doi:10.4244/EIJV9I7A139.
22. Meissner OA, Rieber J, Babaryka G, Oswald M, Reim S, Siebert U, Redel T, Reiser M, Mueller-Lisse U. Intravascular optical coherence tomography: comparison with histopathology in atherosclerotic peripheral artery specimens. J Vasc Interv Radiol. 2006;17:343–9.

23. Brezinski ME, Tearney GJ, Weissman NJ, Boppart SA, Bouma BE, Hee MR, Weyman AE, Swanson EA, Southern JF, Fujimoto JG. Assessing atherosclerotic plaque morphology: comparison of optical coherence tomography and high frequency intravascular ultrasound. Heart. 1997;77:397–403.

24. Shin SH, Baril D, Chaer R, Rhee R, Makaroun M, Marone L. Limitations of the outback LTD re-entry device in femoropopliteal chronic total occlusions. J Vasc Surg. 2011;53(5):1260–4. doi:10.1016/j.jvs.2010.10.127. Epub 2011 Jan 7.

25. Aslam MS, Allaqaband S, Haddadian B, Mori N, Bajwa T, Mewissen M. Subintimal angioplasty with a true reentry device for treatment of chronic total occlusion of the arteries of the lower extremity. Catheter Cardiovasc Interv. 2013;82(5):701–6. doi:10.1002/ccd.22743. Epub 2013 Mar 28.

26. Beschorner U, Sixt S, Schwarzwälder U, Rastan A, Mayer C, Noory E, Macharzina R, Buergelin K, Bonvini R, Zeller T. Recanalization of chronic occlusions of the superficial femoral artery using the Outback re-entry catheter: a single centre experience. Catheter Cardiovasc Interv. 2009;74(6):934–8. doi:10.1002/ccd.22130.

27. Gandini R, Fabiano S, Spano S, Volpi T, Morosetti D, Chiaravalloti A, Nano G, Simonetti G. Randomized control study of the outback LTD reentry catheter versus manual reentry for the treatment of chronic total occlusions in the superficial femoral artery. Catheter Cardiovasc Interv. 2013;82(3):485–92. doi:10.1002/ccd.24742. Epub 2013 Mar 14.

28. Scheinert D, Bräunlich S, Scheinert S, Ulrich M, Biamino G, Schmidt A. Initial clinical experience with an IVUS-guided transmembrane puncture device to facilitate recanalization of total femoral artery occlusions. EuroIntervention. 2005;1(1):115–9.

29. Schmidt A, Keirse K, Blessing E, Langhoff R, Diaz-Cartelle J, European Study Group. Offroad re-entry catheter system for subintimal recanalization of chronic total occlusions in femoropopliteal arteries: primary safety and effectiveness results of the re-route trial. J Cardiovasc Surg. 2014;55(4):551–8. Epub 2014 Jun 13.

30. Scott EC, Biuckians A, Light RE, et al. Subintimal angioplasty for the treatment of claudication and critical limb ischemia: 3- year results. J Vasc Surg. 2007;46:959–64.

31. Flørenes T, Bay D, Sandbaek G, et al. Subintimal angioplasty in the treatment of patients with intermittent claudication: long term results. Eur J Vasc Endovasc Surg. 2004;28:645–50.

32. Met R, Van Lienden KP, Koelemay MJ, et al. Subintimal angioplasty for peripheral arterial occlusive disease: a systematic review. Cardiovasc Intervent Radiol. 2008;31:687–97.

33. Tatli E, Buturak A, Kayapınar O, et al. Subintimal angioplasty and stenting for chronic total femoropopliteal artery occlusions: Early and mid-term outcomes. Cardiol J. 2014; doi:10.5603/CJ.a2014.0043. [Epub ahead of print].

34. Spiliopoulos S, Theodosiadou V, Koukounas V, et al. Distal macro- and microembolization during subintimal recanalization of femoropopliteal chronic total occlusions. J Endovasc Ther. 2014;21:474–81.

35. Hong SJ, Ko YG, Kim JS, Hong MK, Jang Y, Choi D. Midterm outcomes of subintimal angioplasty supported by primary proximal stenting for chronic total occlusion of the superficial femoral artery. J Endovasc Ther. 2013;20:782–91.

36. Jenssen EK, Brosstad F, Pedersen T, et al. Thrombin generation and platelet activation related to subintimal percutaneous transluminal angioplasty. Scand J Clin Lab Invest. 2012;72:23–8.

37. Kitrou P, Parthipun A, Diamantopoulous A, et al. Targeted true lumen re-entry with the Outback catheter: accuracy, success and complications in 100 peripheral chronic total occlusions and systemic review of the literature. J Endovasc Ther. 2015;22:538–45.

38. Final Results Presented for Covidien's PFAST-CTO Study, 2012. http://evtoday.com/2012/10/final-results-presented-for-covidiens-pfast-ctosstudy.

39. Sethi S, Mohammad A, Ahmed SH, et al. Recanalization of popliteal and infrapopliteal chronic total occlusions using Viance and CrossBoss crossing catheters: a multicenter experience from the XL-PAD Registry. J Invasive Cardiol. 2015;27(1):2–7.

Chapter 7
Complications of Peripheral Arterial Interventions

Mazen Abu-Fadel

7.1 Introduction

Atherosclerotic disease remains the most common cause of death in the Western world. Data from population studies have demonstrated an increased prevalence of peripheral arterial disease (PAD) in patients older than 40 years of age. In the current era of advanced endovascular equipment, techniques and expertise in PAD interventions, percutaneous interventions on aortoiliac, and femoropopliteal and infrapopliteal disease have increased significantly with very favorable outcomes compared to surgical revascularization. Complications from such procedures can be both life and limb threatening. Timely diagnosis and managment of complications is crutial to prevent unfavorable outcomes. This chapter sumarizes the complications most likely seen in peripheral arterial interventions and discusses dianostic and theraputic approaches to treat them.

In patients undergoing endovascular therapy for symptomatic PAD, 60% of diabetics and 30% of nondiabetics will have a chronic total occlusion (CTO) of at least one arterial bed of the lower extremities [1]. It has become evident that endovascular management of femoropopliteal lesions even CTOs results in good primary and secondary patency at 2 years. This therapy should be considered as first-line option for many patients with peripheral artery disease, including those with critical limb ischemia, claudication with poor bypass conduit, or patients at high medical risk for open surgical revascularization [2]. Such percutaneous approaches have become the treatment of choice for the majority of patients presenting with atherosclerotic PAD. Complications of endovascular procedures, although infrequent, can occur in

M. Abu-Fadel, MD, FACC, FSCAI
Associate Professor of Medicine, Vice Chief, Section of Cardiovascular Medicine Director, Interventional Cardiology & Cardiac Cath Lab Program Director, Interventional Cardiology Fellowship University of Oklahoma HScC, Oklahoma City, OK, USA
e-mail: mazen-abufadel@ouhsc.edu

© Springer Science+Business Media Singapore 2017
S. Banerjee (ed.), *Practical Approach to Peripheral Arterial Chronic Total Occlusions*, DOI 10.1007/978-981-10-3053-6_7

as many as 5–8% of endovascular procedures and may result in significant disability including limb loss and death. This chapter will review the most commonly encountered complications including access site complications, perforations/ruptures, dissections, and distal embolization.

7.2 Arterial Access for Endovascular Interventions

Access site complications remain the most encountered complication of any diagnostic or interventional procedure. Such complications were much more frequent in the early years of endovascular interventions due to the need for larger introducer sheaths (9–10 F). More recently, improved technology and specialized equipment have allowed the interventionalist to perform more complex procedures through smaller sheaths and alternate access routes such as radial, brachial, popliteal, and pedal arteries. However, the common femoral artery (CFA) remains the most commonly used artery for endovascular interventions. Multiple factors increase the risk of complications after vascular access. These factors are divided into modifiable or non-modifiable risk factors or, more commonly, into patient- or procedure-related factors. Patient-related factors include patients' sex, age, body mass index, compliance with bed rest, and the presence of chronic diseases such as hypertension and renal dysfunction. Procedure-related factors include operator experience, faulty access technique including venous punctures or multiple arterial punctures, suboptimal arteriotomy site, sheath size, sheath dwell time, and periprocedural medications including thrombolytic, anticoagulation, and antiplatelet agents.

The first and most important step in avoiding access site complications is to use meticulous technique to obtain access into the arterial circulation. Ideally, the CFA should be accessed below the most inferior border of the inferior epigastric artery (IEA) and above the CFA bifurcation into the profunda and superficial femoral arteries (Fig. 7.1). In 35% of patients, the bifurcation of the CFA occurs below the inferior border of the femoral head [3]. This segment of the CFA from the inferior border of the femoral head to the bifurcation should also be avoided since this part of the CFA cannot be easily compressed against the head of the femur to achieve hemostasis. Access below the CFA bifurcation or the inferior border of the femoral head – whichever of these landmarks is more cranial – will result in an increased risk of hematomas and pseudoaneurysms. On the other hand, access above the most inferior border of the (IEA) will increase the risk of retroperitoneal hemorrhage which may be fatal [4]. In light of these considerations, the ideal access site into the CFA lies at or just above the middle of the head of the femur (Fig. 7.1) [5]. If a previous angiogram of the access site is available, it is very important to review it prior to attempting access into the same CFA to determine the location of the inferior epigastric artery and bifurcation into profunda and SFA arteries to ideal the optimal site for atrial access. If this is not available, appropriate techniques should be used to ensure an ideal puncture site into the CFA.

Fig. 7.1 Access site angiogram showing the ideal arteriotomy site over the midline of the femoral head (*star*). The lowermost deflection of the inferior epigastric artery (*IEA*) is shown (*white arrow*) as well as the common femoral artery bifurcation (*black arrow*)

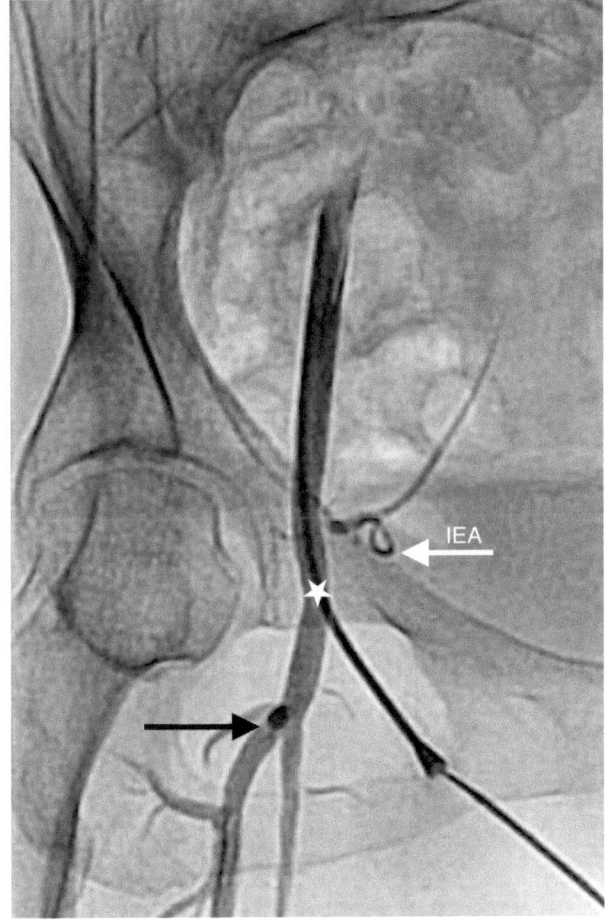

Fluoroscopy guidance may help in improving access into the CFA. In general, fluoroscopy may be used in two different ways. The first is the indirect fluoroscopy technique where a metallic object such as the tip of a hemostat can be used to locate the inferior border of the femoral head under fluoroscopy in the posterior-anterior projection with no cranial or caudal angulation. Access to the CFA can then be achieved by advancing the needle from that landmark toward the CFA. It has been shown that this technique does not increase the success rate of cannulating the CFA but it does significantly decrease arteriotomies below the most inferior border of the head of the femur [3]. The reason why indirect fluoroscopy is not always helpful has to do with the fact that the amount of subcutaneous tissue that the needle has to traverse before entering the CFA is variable from patient to another and thus the arteriotomy site will be variable. In addition, this technique will not help locate the CFA bifurcation prior to sheath insertion.

On the other hand, the direct fluoroscopy technique requires repetitive fluoroscopy of the access site with low-dose fluoro in the posterior-anterior projection with every needle advancement until access is established at the desired level. This technique is best done with a micropuncture needle. After locating the inferior border of the femoral head, repeat fluoroscopy is performed after the needle has been advanced into the subcutaneous tissue but has not entered the CFA. This will help the operator guide the tip of the needle toward the middle of the femoral head to achieve an ideal puncture site. This method will increase the radiation exposure to the patient and to a certain extent to the operator. It is crucial to keep fluoroscopy use to a minimum. In addition, the bifurcation of the CFA is also not identified prior to access and imaging of the site with angiography [6]. When using a micropuncture needle, the operator should follow the wire into the iliac circulation and the distal aorta under fluoroscopy since the 0.018″ wire may travel into small branches (Fig. 7.2) and cause a wire perforation that may lead to retroperitoneal hemorrhage [7]. Prior to inserting the procedural sheath, a femoral angiogram should be done using the micropuncture sheath dilator. It is best to do the angiogram by attaching the sheath dilator to a pressure transducer prior to injecting through it to make sure it is in the true lumen and not against the vessel wall to avoid dissections and perforations. After angiography, if the access site is not in an ideal location, the dilator can be removed and manual pressure held for 3–5 min and access reattempted now that there is a femoral angiogram to guide access into the CFA. It is important to mention that injecting through the micropuncture dilator has a risk of iliac artery dissection especially in tortuous arteries.

Without a previous angiogram for CFA access, fluoroscopy cannot always identify the optimal access site due to the anatomic variation in the CFA and its bifurcation. Ultrasound-guided access has emerged as a superior technique and has multiple advantages over fluoroscopy. The ultrasound image will allow the operator to directly visualize the CFA and its bifurcation. In some patients, it may also show the inguinal ligament. In addition, the needle can be directed in real time toward the anterior wall of the CFA and can be seen going through the anterior wall of the CFA but not the posterior wall. Disease and calcifications in the CFA can also be seen and avoided. Ultrasound-guided access has been shown in a multicenter randomized controlled trial to improve CFA cannulation in patients with high CFA bifurcations. It also reduced the number of attempts to obtain access, decreased the total time to sheath insertion, and decreased the risk of venipuncture. In addition, ultrasound guidance significantly decreased access site complications (1.4% vs. 3.4%, $p = 0.04$), a finding that was driven by reductions in access-site hematomas [8].

Advancements in percutaneous technologies have resulted >90% technical success rates in peripheral interventions. As such, interventionalists have begun to tackle and treat more complex disease that would have been traditionally treated with surgery or more conservative measures. For these reasons, situations arise in which alternative access sites are needed to successfully perform femoropopliteal and infrapopliteal interventions, especially chronic total occlusions. Popliteal

Fig. 7.2 Access with micropuncture needle and wire. After resistance was encountered, fluoroscopy showed the wire in a pelvic branch (*arrow*) instead of going into the iliac system through the common iliac artery stent (*star*)

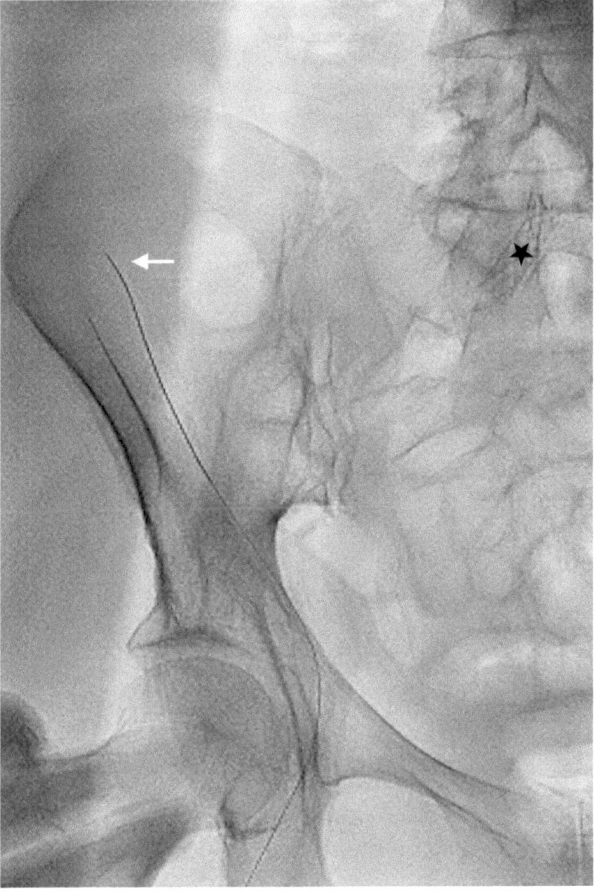

artery access is attractive because it supports 5–7F sheaths and provides support for retrograde crossing, and balloons/stents can be deployed. The success rate of popliteal access is >90% and almost 100% if ultrasound guidance is used. In an effort to decrease vascular complications, it has been recommended to screen patients with ultrasonography and exclude those with heavy calcifications of the popliteal artery or those with popliteal aneurysms [9]. A micropuncture needle is also recommended especially the echogenic tip needle that may be used more easily with ultrasound. The most common access-related complications of the popliteal artery included popliteal artery hematomas, AV fistulae, and pseudoaneurysms (Figs. 7.3 and 7.4).

Pedal access may be very helpful in recanalizing the popliteal and infrapopliteal arteries, particularly in patients with critical limb ischemia as the disease is usually lengthy, calcific, and occlusive. It is best to assess the pedal arteries with ultrasound prior to the procedure, or if an antegrade sheath is present in the common femoral

Fig. 7.3 Color Doppler ultrasound of the popliteal artery showing an AV fistula as a complication of popliteal artery access for intervention on a totally occluded superficial femoral artery

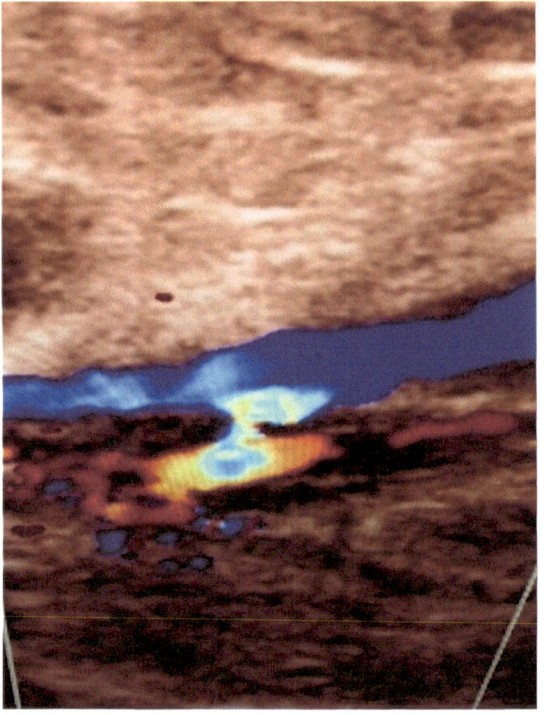

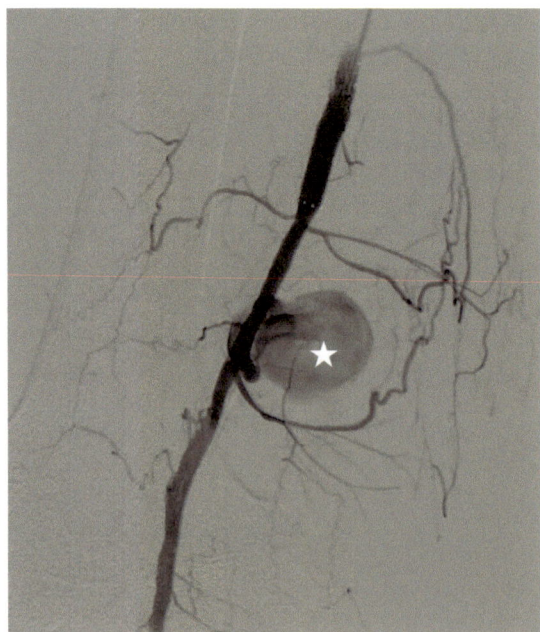

Fig. 7.4 Angiogram demonstrating a large pseudoaneurysm (*star*) in the proximal popliteal artery 2 weeks after accessing this artery for an intervention on a totally occluded superficial femoral artery. This was successfully treated with a self-expanding covered stent

Fig. 7.5 Bleeding from
wire perforation after
diagnostic angiogram from
the radial artery causing
compartmental syndrome
requiring fasciotomy

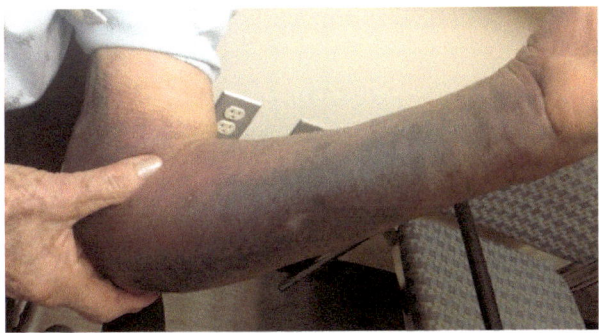

or popliteal arteries, antegrade contrast injections with direct arterial puncture under fluoroscopy can be done. Complications include hematoma and rarely dissection, compartment syndrome, thrombosis, and occlusion of the vessel which may be catastrophic in some cases [10].

Brachial and radial access may be used for aortoiliac, CFA, and proximal superficial femoral artery interventions. The brachial artery may be more prone to complications. Thus, the radial artery is more commonly used. The risk of bleeding from the radial artery is small compared to other vascular beds. More frequent and serious complications include radial artery occlusion reported to occur in up to 4% of patients. Patent hemostasis has been shown to reduce the risk of radial artery occlusion to 1% [11]. Pseudoaneurysms are uncommon in the radial artery but may occur and present late. The treatment is with ultrasound-guided compression, thrombin injection, or surgery. Moreover, wires or catheters may cause perforation along the radial artery or any of its side branches. The incidence is reported to be 0.01% [12]. If the perforated segment of the radial artery can be or is already crossed with a wire, continuing with the procedure while the sheath or guide catheter covers the perforation site may help seal the perforation. An angiogram of the artery at the end of the case should be performed to confirm that the perforation has been sealed. If the segment cannot be crossed, applying a pressure dressing or inflating a blood pressure cuff along the course of the radial artery will often seal the leak. Compartment syndrome is rare and has been reported to occur in 0.004% of patients in one large case series [13] (Fig. 7.5).

7.3 Access Site-Related Complications

Even after ideal arterial access using all available techniques and equipment by the most experienced operators, access site complications and bleeding may still occur after sheath removal or closure device deployment. While all access-related complications are serious and important, in this chapter, we shall briefly discuss some of the more serious complications associated with vascular access.

7.3.1 Pseudoaneurysms

A pseudoaneurysm (PSA) occurs when an arterial puncture site does not adequately seal and causes a contained rupture with disruption in all three layers of the arterial wall. Pulsatile blood leaving the artery into the perivascular space causes a hematoma that then forms the wall of the PSA. The incidence of PSA after diagnostic angiograms can be as high as 2%. This number may reach up to 8% following peripheral interventions and probably relates to the presence of more common femoral disease as well as risk factors that are associated with more difficult hemostasis (e.g., ESRD, DM) [14, 15]. PSAs usually present as pain and swelling at the access site. Large PSAs may cause local compression of the structures in the femoral sheath leading to neuropathy, deep thrombosis, claudication, or, rarely, critical limb ischemia. Subjectively, the patient will experience groin pain disproportionate to the physical findings including a palpable pulsatile mass or the presence of a systolic bruit. There may also be skin ischemia and necrosis if the PSA is large and tense. The diagnostic test of choice is Doppler ultrasonography of the access site that has 94% sensitivity and 97% specificity to identify a PSA (Fig. 7.6).

Different therapeutic strategies have been validated to treat PSA, including simple manual compression, ultrasound-guided compression, and ultrasound-guided thrombin injection. In general, if the PSA is <10 mm, most will resolve spontaneously with no intervention. It is recommended to follow them with ultrasound on a biweekly basis until resolution. A treatment algorithm based on the morphological

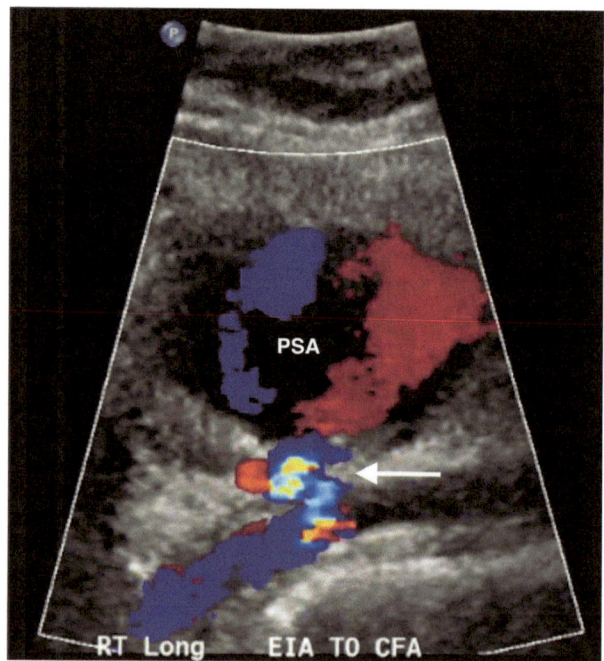

Fig. 7.6 Color Doppler ultrasound showing a pseudoaneurysm (*PSA*) at the common femoral artery access site with a narrow neck (*arrow*) and to-and-fro blood flow in the PSA

features of PSA has been developed, evaluated, and published by Dzijan-Horn et al., which has resulted in an overall PSA treatment success rate of 97.2% with an acceptable complication rate of 1.5% [16]. According to the algorithm, small PSAs (diameter <20 mm), PSAs without clearly definable neck, PSAs directly adjacent to vessels, and PSAs with concomitant arteriovenous fistula were treated by manual compression. On the other hand, large PSAs and those with definable neck and away from the vessels and with no arteriovenous fistula were treated by ultrasound-guided thrombin injection. There were few patients who crossed over between manual compression and thrombin injection. When followed, the treatment algorithm for post-procedural PSAs was not successful in 12 of 428 patients (2.8%). Ten of these patients required surgical repair, which by itself had a 30% complication rate. The other two patients required covered stents to exclude the PSA. It is thus recommended that even in case of initial treatment failure, it is worth performing further attempts according to this algorithm before escalating therapy toward surgical repair [16]. In other series, surgical repair of PSA was reported to have complication rates as high as 60–70%. In the current era, surgical repair is left as a last resort of treatment for PSAs and mainly done in the setting of failure of percutaneous intervention, rapid expansion of PSAs, recurrence, skin necrosis, nerve palsy, limb ischemia, and infected (mycotic) PSAs.

Ultrasound-guided compression involves the location of the PSA neck with ultrasound and then applying pressure with the ultrasound probe directly over the neck to completely occlude the flow into and out of the PSA. Pressure is applied initially for 20–25 min, after which more pressure may be applied if the flow is still seen with Doppler ultrasound. Applying direct pressure is usually painful for the patient, and sedation or pain control should be given prior to staring the compression. A follow-up ultrasound is usually performed at 24 h and 1 week to confirm that the PSA remains closed. Some of the risks associated with this technique involve distal embolization of the thrombin material into the arterial circulation. The severity of the complication will vary, but most of these patients will require urgent angiography for diagnostic purposes and intervention as deemed clinically necessary.

Ultrasound-guided thrombin injection is done if compression of the neck fails to occlude the PSA and it involved visualizing the PSA under Doppler ultrasound and injecting under direct visualization thrombin into the PSA sac. The amount of thrombin injected may vary from patient to patient, and it is best to inject just enough thrombin in the base of the PSA away from the neck slowly over 10–15 min until there is cessation of color flow by Doppler in the PSA. Patients are kept on bed rest for at least 6 h, and a follow-up Doppler is done at 24 h and 1 week post-procedure. A multiloculated PSA may require thrombin injection into its different lobes to assure complete resolution. There are some reports of applying balloon occlusion at low pressures of the feeding artery while injecting the PSA with thrombin. This is usually done when the neck of the PSA is short or >5 mm in diameter by ultrasound. This technique may decrease the risk of distal embolization of thrombin into the circulation and the risk of iatrogenic limb ischemia. Other reported ways to occlude PSA include coil embolization and covered stenting of the feeding artery (Fig. 7.7a, b).

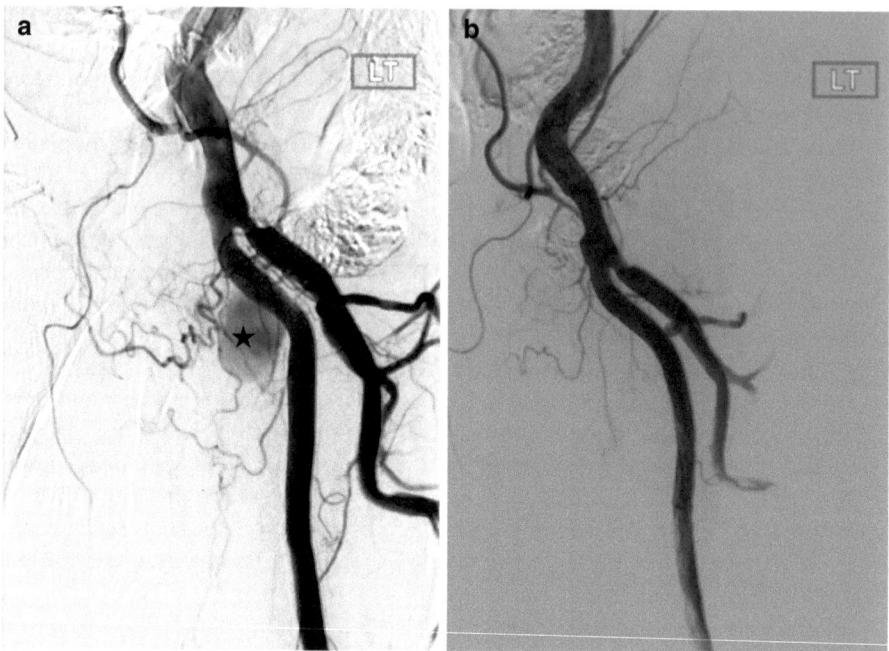

Fig. 7.7 (**a**) Shows a pseudoaneurysm (*star*) in the proximal portion of the superficial femoral artery (SFA) that was caused due to a low femoral arteriotomy below the femoral head and the CFA bifurcation. This was treated successfully with a self-expanding covered stent (**b**)

7.3.2 Retroperitoneal Hemorrhage

Retroperitoneal hemorrhage (RPH) is the most life-threatening complication seen with femoral-based access. The incidence of retroperitoneal hemorrhage in vascular access-related complications is between 0.15% and 0.44% [17]. The retroperitoneal space can accommodate a very large volume of blood even before any clinical symptoms such as hypotension and tachycardia arise. Up to three-fourths of patients with RPH receive blood transfusions, and mortality may be as high as 10%. Predictors of development of a retroperitoneal bleed in the setting of peripheral interventions included low body weight, Angioseal device use, sheath placement above the inferior epigastric artery, female sex, use of IIb/IIIa inhibitors, and larger sheath size [4]. Most often, patient starts showing symptoms early after the procedure, but sometimes RPH may present much later. Patient can experience mild to severe lower back and flank pain most often on the same side as the access site. They may also complain of vague abdominal pain and distension. There is usually no obvious sign of swelling or a hematoma at the puncture site with this form of hemorrhage. As patients continue to bleed into the retroperitoneal space, tachycardia and hypotension will develop followed by shock. A decrease in hemoglobin and hematocrit may become evident soon after. It is important to remember that hemodynamic compromise is usually a late sign of retroperitoneal hemorrhage, and if it is suspected, early aggressive resuscitation measures are important. While the gold standard for diagnosing retroperitoneal hemorrhage is computed tomography (CT) of the abdomen and pelvis, this should be done only if the patient is stable enough to be transferred to the radiology suite. Clinical diagnosis and rapid management remain the most important and lifesaving intervention. Two large IV lines should be established, and blood should be prepared and kept on standby. IV fluids should be given rapidly until blood is available. Manual pressure should be applied to the access site even in the absence of a hematoma since sometimes the arteriotomy is in a compressible location. Anticoagulation medication should be held if possible, and surgical evaluation should be sought depending on the severity of retroperitoneal hemorrhage and, if it is ongoing, causing hemodynamic compromise [18]. Intervention should be performed on patients with refractory hypotension or on patients with an active blush on computed tomography. Either surgical repair or endovascular balloon tamponade or exclusion with a covered stent can be performed [19]. If during femoral angiography the sheath is noted to be high, off-label use of suture-mediated closure devices for arteriotomies above the most inferior defection of the inferior epigastric artery and contralateral access with balloon tamponade (and covered stenting if needed) have been reported and utilized as a preventive measure to avoid RPH in high-risk patients.

7.3.3   Arteriovenous Fistula Formation

Throughout the body, arteries and veins are closely associated and paired with each other. As such any faulty instrumentation of one of the structures may lead a communication between the artery and vein causing and acquired arteriovenous fistula (AVF). In case of endovascular procedures, AVF is a communication between the artery and vein at the access site that cause a continuous flow of arterial blood into the venous system (Figs. 7.3 and 7.8). This is most commonly caused by lateral or medial needle deviation or needle placement during access leading to combined arterial and venous puncture. If the sheath is placed, the communication will get larger and may lead to AVF in the right setting. Another important factor is accessing both the common femoral artery and vein at the same level and not holding adequate pressure for hemostasis. This may cause a communication between the two structures the lead to an AVF. Although less common, iatrogenic AVF can result from devices used in peripheral and venous interventions such as endovenous laser for saphenous ablation, percutaneous directional atherectomy, and devices used for reentry during subintimal angioplasty.

In most cases, the communication is small and seals off spontaneously. However, in some patients with increased risk such as older patients, females, patients with high body mass index, patients with hypertension, those receiving anticoagulation or antifibrinolytic therapy, or those undergoing left-sided access, low or multiple needle punctures are at higher risk of acquiring an AVF [20, 21]. While this is

Fig. 7.8 Distal aortography with bilateral iliofemoral angiography showing a left arteriovenous fistulae (AVF) at the level of the superficial femoral artery in a patient not known to have peripheral arterial disease previously and not known to have the AVF

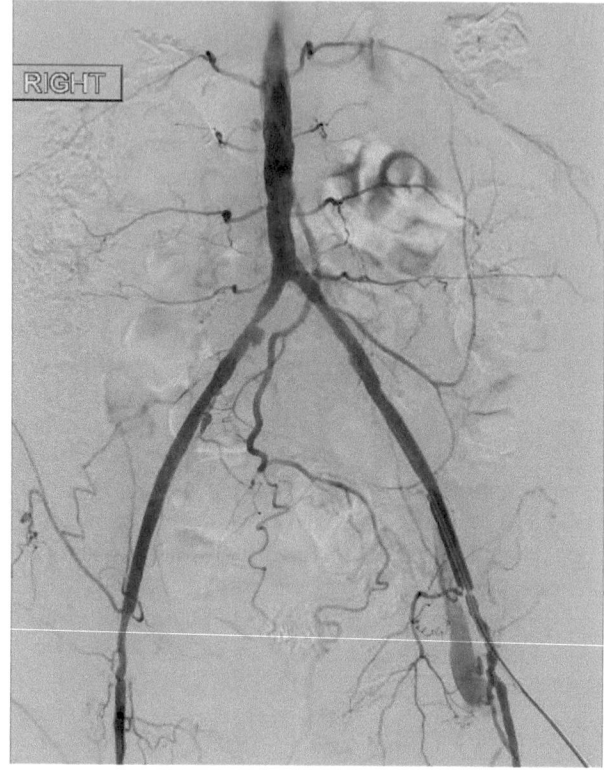

usually painless, a thrill and/or a bruit could be felt/heard on physical exam of the groin. Long-standing AVFs can lead to limb edema or ischemia due to steal, high-output cardiac failure, or aneurysmal degeneration of the artery [22]. Duplex ultrasound is the diagnostic test of choice for evaluating patients with suspected AVFs. Angiography may be needed in some cases. Some of the AVFs are also diagnosed incidentally when a patient presents for repeat angiography.

Treatment options depend on the size and the symptoms associated with the AVF. In general, most small, asymptomatic AVFs will thrombose spontaneously. In those causing symptoms, surgery remains the gold standard, but other modalities are being used more frequently including ultrasound-guided compression and endovascular interventions if feasible. Unlike with PSAs, ultrasound-guided compression of AVFs is not as effective in obliterating the AVF especially if it has been present for over 2 weeks or the patient is on anticoagulation [23]. In general the procedure is successful in up to about 30% of patients. Compression is done for at least 10 min under direct visualization and without compromising distal flow into the extremity. This is usually a painful procedure; therefore, the use of sedation or pain medication is recommended. For those patient who develop symptoms due to AVF, including edema of the lower extremity, ischemia, high-output heart failure, or progressive enlargement of the AVF with increase in shunting or recurrence after conservative management, it is recommended that they undergo repair either surgical or endovascular. Covered stent placement or embolization techniques may be effective as an alternative to surgical repair for high-risk patients. However, the use of stents depends upon the location of the fistula. In general covered stents are best avoided in the common femoral artery but may be a good choice in the superficial femoral artery.

7.3.4 Other Access Site-Related Complications

Other access site-related complications include hematomas, dissections, arterial occlusions, infections, and others. Table 7.1 presents a brief discussion about these complications. The utilization of the radial artery for some peripheral interventions has allowed early ambulation and fewer access site-bleeding complications. In addition, while this access site is not suitable for all patients, it may provide an easier intervention in some anatomical situations [24]. Equipment size and shaft length may prohibit the use of the radial artery in many peripheral interventions especially in the distal lower extremity vascular beds.

Vascular closure devices seem to be at least non-inferior to manual compression and in real-life registry data even superior in decreasing vascular access site complications. However, these devices seem to have a set of complications that are specific to them, and care should be taken on whom they should be used. Screening with femoral angiography while or directly after obtaining femoral artery access and avoiding the use of anticoagulation in patients with high or low arteriotomies as well as the avoidance of vascular closure devices in the presence of puncture site-related risk factors might reduce the risk of vascular complications.

7.4 Anticoagulation Use-Related Complications

The use of bivalirudin vs. unfractionated heparin (UFH) in patients undergoing endovascular peripheral interventions (EPI) has been reported in several studies. Some of these studies have suggested that bivalirudin offers the same efficacy as UFH but with reduced bleeding complication rates [25]. However, a meta-analysis that included a total of 1249 patients enrolled in four nonrandomized clinical trials comparing UFH to bivalirudin showed that there was no significant difference between the two arms in terms of total bleeding complications (RR 0.64, 95% CI 0.31–1.34). Similarly, no difference was observed in terms of major bleed (RR 0.58, 95% CI 0.2–1.65) or minor bleed (RR 0.66, 95% CI 0.38–1.61) [26].

Table 7.1 Modified from Critical Care Nurse Vol 32, No. 5, OCTOBER 2012

Complication	Description	Clinical findings	Management
Hematoma Incidence: 5–23%	The most common vascular access site complication. A collection of blood located in the soft tissue. May occur if the arterial puncture is below the inferior boarder of the femoral head or below the CFA bifurcation	Visible swelling surrounding the puncture site. Area of hardening under the skin surrounding the puncture site that will vary in size. Often associated with pain in the groin area that can occur at rest or with leg movement. Can result in decrease in hemoglobin and blood pressure and increase in heart rate, depending on severity	Apply pressure to site. Mark the area to evaluate for any change in size. If large, monitor serial blood cell counts and give IV fluids. Maintain/prolong bed rest. Interrupt anticoagulant and antiplatelet medications if needed, and transfuse blood if indicated. If severe, may require surgical evacuation. Many hematomas resolve within a few weeks as the blood dissipates and is absorbed into the tissue
Retroperitoneal hemorrhage Incidence: 0.15–0.44%	Bleeding that occurs behind the serous membrane lining the walls of the abdomen and pelvis. May occur if the arterial wall puncture is made above the inguinal ligament, resulting in perforation of the external iliac artery or penetration of the posterior wall. Can be fatal if not recognized early	Moderate to severe and sometimes vague abdominal or back pain. Ipsilateral flank pain. Ecchymosis and decrease in hemoglobin and hematocrit are late signs. Abdominal distention. Often not associated with obvious swelling or hematoma. Hypotension and tachycardia. Diagnosed clinically and confirmed by computed tomography or angiography	Two large bore intravenous lines for intravenous fluid resuscitation. Perform serial blood cell counts. Maintain/prolong bed rest. Interrupt anticoagulant and antiplatelet medications. Blood transfusion, if indicated. If severe, may require surgical evacuation or endovascular treatment in the catheterization lab

(continued)

Table 7.1 (continued)

Complication	Description	Clinical findings	Management
Pseudoaneurysm Incidence: 0.5–9%	A communicating tract between the tissue and, usually, one of the weaker walls of the femoral artery, causing blood to escape from the artery into the surrounding tissue. Possible causes include difficulty with arterial cannulation, inadequate compression after sheath removal, and impaired hemostasis. May occur if the arterial puncture is below the inferior boarder of the femoral head or below the CFA bifurcation	Swelling at insertion site. Large, painful hematoma. Ecchymosis. Pulsatile mass. Bruit and/or thrill in the groin. Pseudoaneurysms can rupture, causing abrupt swelling and severe pain. Suspect nerve compression when pain is out of proportion to size of hematoma. Nerve compression can result in limb weakness that takes weeks or months to resolve. Diagnosed by ultrasound	Maintain/prolong bed rest. Small femoral pseudoaneurysms should be monitored; they commonly close spontaneously after cessation of anticoagulant therapy. Large femoral pseudoaneurysms can be treated by ultrasound-guided compression, surgical intervention, or ultrasound-guided thrombin injection
Arteriovenous fistula Incidence: 0.2–2.1%	A direct communication between an artery and a vein that occurs when the artery and vein are punctured. The communication occurs once the sheath is removed. Risk factors: Multiple access attempts Punctures above or below ideal CFA site Impaired clotting mechanisms	Can be asymptomatic. Bruit and/or thrill at access site. Swollen, tender extremity. Distal arterial insufficiency and/or deep venous thrombosis can result in limb ischemia. Congestive heart failure. Confirmed by ultrasound	Some arteriovenous fistulae resolve spontaneously without intervention. Some arteriovenous fistulae require ultrasound-guided compression or surgical repair

(continued)

Table 7.1 (continued)

Complication	Description	Clinical findings	Management
Arterial occlusion Incidence: <0.8–20%	Occlusion of an artery by a thromboembolism. Most common sources: mural thrombus originating in cardiac chambers, vascular aneurysms, or vascular atherosclerotic plaques. Thromboemboli can develop at sheath site or catheter tip; embolization occurs during sheath removal. Prevention or at least reduction can be obtained by anticoagulation, vasodilators, and nursing vigilance	Classic symptoms include the 5 Ps: Pain Paralysis Paresthesias Pulselessness Pallor Doppler studies help localize the area. Angiogram is required to identify exact location of occlusion site	Treatment depends on size/type of embolus, location, and patient's ability to tolerate ischemia in affected area. Small thromboemboli in well-perfused arterial areas may undergo spontaneous lysis. Larger thromboemboli may require thromboembolectomy, surgery, and/or thrombolytic agents. Distal embolic protection devices (i.e., filters) may be placed if necessary
Femoral neuropathy Incidence: 0.21–23%	Nerve damage caused by injury of the femoral nerve(s) during access and/or compression of nerves by a hematoma	Pain and/or tingling at femoral access site. Numbness at access site or further down the leg. Leg weakness. Difficulty moving the affected leg. Decreased patellar tendon reflex	Identification and treatment of the source. Treatment of symptoms. Physical therapy
Infection Incidence: <0.1–20%	Colonization by a pathogen Causes: compromised technique, poor hygiene, prolonged indwelling sheath time. Femoral access closure device	Pain, erythema, swelling at access site with possible purulent discharge. Fever Increased white blood cell count	Symptomatic treatment for pain. Antibiotics. Surgical removal of foreign body such as closure device if necessary

7.5 Procedural-Related Complications

Peripheral complications include but are not limited to arterial dissections, vessel occlusions, perforations, and distal embolization. The incidence of these complications, while low in general, is higher in patients undergoing recanalization of chronic total occlusions than for stenotic vessels. Analysis of a large national database of patients undergoing peripheral interventions shows the overall complication rate to be 14.46%. These complications were noted to be significantly lower (13.36%) in high-volume centers (fourth quartile with >126 peripheral interventions/year) as compared to the lowest-quartile-volume centers (≤36 cases/year) with a complication rate of 15.66% ($p < 0.001$). Similarly, the in-hospital mortality, amputation rate, and vascular complications were all significantly lower in the highest-volume centers compared to the lowest-volume ones [27]. In addition, a multivariate analysis revealed age, female gender, and baseline comorbidities to be significant predictors of mortality. Emergent/urgent procedures as well as weekend admissions also predicted higher complication rates and worst outcomes [27].

Perhaps the most appropriate method to manage complications is to avoid them. Since this is not always possible, it is of utmost importance for any interventionalist to be familiar with diagnosing and treating complications associated with peripheral interventions. Preprocedural planning and knowing each patients anatomy are crucial to determine if and what endovascular strategy is possible and to help decrease complication rates. For CTO interventions, the proximal and distal level of the occlusion and the pattern of the collateral circulation should be assessed to help in choosing what strategy and approach to take during the intervention. These strategies may include access site, retrograde vs. antegrade approach to cross the occlusion, and how to best avoid severing collateral flow, which may lead to worsening ischemia if revascularization is not achieved during the same setting.

7.5.1 Perforations

Perforations can occur from a variety of causes. Most commonly they are due to wire perforations; however, balloon angioplasty-, stenting-, or atherectomy-related perforations are also common. If unrecognized or not managed appropriately, they may result in significant morbidity and even mortality [28]. The most important factors of patient outcomes are the location of the perforation and the speed of recognition [29]. Bleeding in the pelvis, abdominal cavity, or thorax is life-threatening, while bleeding in a compartmentalized space such as the arm or leg is usually less severe but may still lead to major morbidity such as compartmental syndrome.

Perforations may be more easily avoided in non-CTO interventions since good angiographic imaging and the use of road maps can help keep wires and devices in the true lumen. In addition, vessel architecture, size, plaque burden, and plaque orientation can be more easily assessed. In CTO interventions, vessel wall calcifications can help guide the operator advance wires in the direction of the vessel architecture and may provide a road map of the vessel lumen. While it would be easy to recognize when the wire traverses outside the calcified vessel wall, if the artery is not calcified, especially in iliac CTO interventions, the operator will need to assess the wire position carefully before proceeding with the intervention [28].

Wire perforations are the most common and usually occur in the distal vascular beds or in small side branches (Fig. 7.9). In general, straight, stiffer, and hydrophilic wires tend to cause more perforations. While some wire perforations may be serious in the coronary of cerebral circulation, in general, wire perforations in the lower extremities are minor and most of the time will seal on their own. Very rarely the operator will need to abandon the procedure or reverse anticoagulation. Most important is to recognize when a guidewire has perforated the vessel to prevent worsening the complication by advancing a larger catheter or performing angioplasty across the perforation. If the perforation does not stop spontaneously, inflating a manual blood pressure cuff around the extremity to above systolic pressures for 3–5 min around the area of perforation can stop the bleeding. This usually works for both main vessel and side branch perforations especially in the SFA circulation. In other cases, balloon tamponade with a low-pressure inflation (2–4 atm) to occlude flow across the perforation or the perforated side branch will be sufficient. Coiling may be the best option especially if the wire perforation is in a small side branch and not responding to conservative measures. Balloon tamponade alone or placement of a covered stent in the SFA to exclude the origin of the side branch may not entirely stop the bleeding because collateral pathways may continue to perfuse the injured vessel [28].

Balloons, stents, and atherectomy devices usually cause larger perforations or vessel tears and ruptures. While these complications are less frequent, they are, in general, more severe (Fig. 7.10a–d). As a rule, larger diameter vessels are more at risk of perforation with stretching than those with smaller vessel diameters. This is important to keep in mind when performing interventions on iliac arteries and distal aorta. When stretched, larger arteries will cause the patient to feel pain, and this should be a sign to refrain from further balloon dilatation or stent expansion. Factors known to increase the risk of perforations during lower extremity interventions include diabetes, older age, and critical limb ischemia [30]. Other factors that may contribute to vessel rupture include CTOs, oversizing of balloons and balloon-expandable stents, high inflation pressures especially in calcified, and difficult to dilate lesions. Even nominal pressure inflations in calcified and totally occluded vessels may lead to perforations. Atherectomy-related perforations happen due to direct shaving or mechanical disruption of the adventitial layer of the vessel wall. Depending on the atherectomy device used, the procedural perforation rate will vary between 0.5% and 5.3% [31–34].

Similar to wire perforations, the outcomes of device-related perforations depend on the severity and location of the complications. Dye extravasation, especially in a

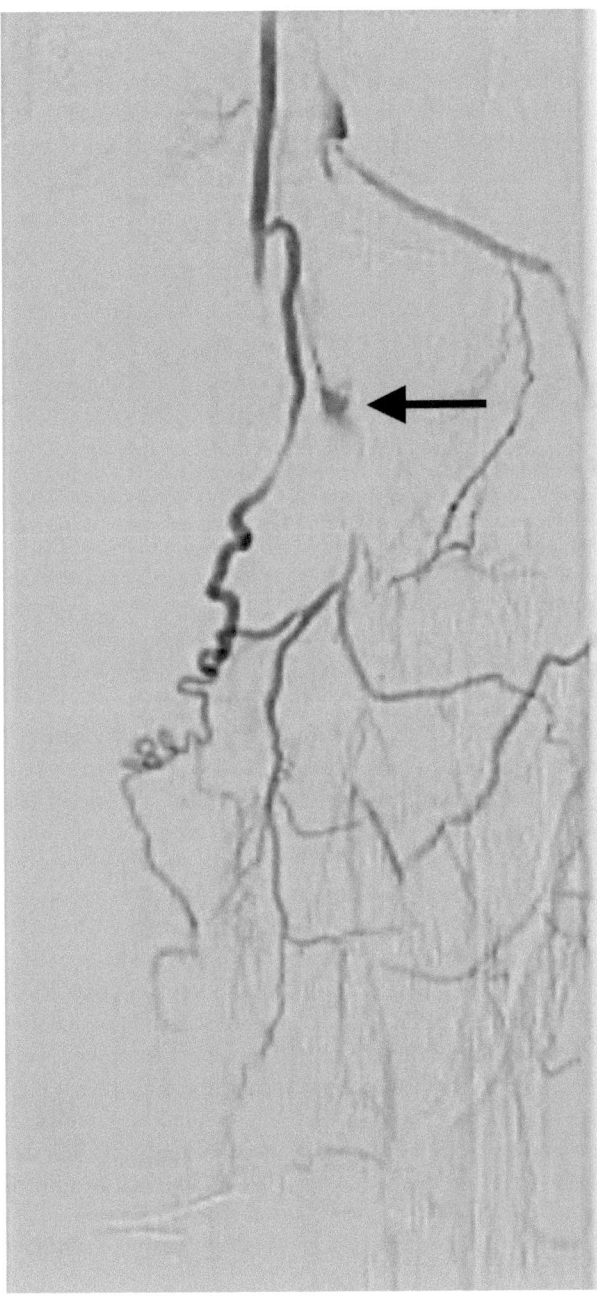

Fig. 7.9 Wire perforation during an intervention on a totally occluded superficial femoral artery. A hydrophilic wire went into a small branch of the collateral and caused the perforation (arrow). The procedure was completed successfully, and anticoagulation was not reversed. The perforation sealed after crossing the SFA and ballooning across the takeoff of the collateral for a minute

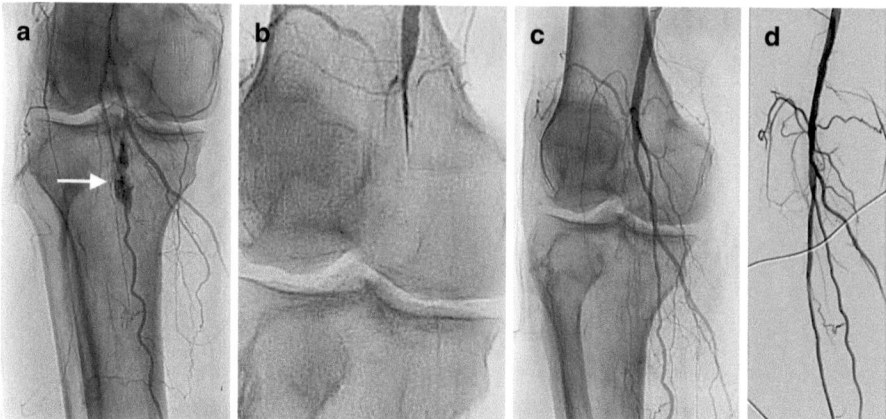

Fig. 7.10 (**a**) Shows a large perforation caused by a chronic total occlusion (CTO) crossing device while attempting to cross a CTO of the popliteal artery. A blood pressure cuff was inflated around the site of perforation for 3 min. While the cuff was inflated, there was no flow to the distal extremity, and the perforation was not bleeding (**b**). After the blood pressure cuff was deflated, repeat angiogram showed resolution of bleeding (**c**). The procedure was completed successfully using a wire and catheter to cross the occlusion successfully and revascularize the popliteal occlusion (**d**)

body cavity such as the pelvis from iliac perforations (Fig 7.11a, b), represents the most severe finding that may lead to hemorrhagic shock and death and should be dealt with promptly. An extravascular blush or stain that persists on fluoroscopy represents a contained perforation that is usually smaller in size. Due to the life-threatening nature of iliac perforations, a 7F sheath is usually recommended for iliac interventions especially CTOs to allow the advancement and deployment of covered stents if needed urgently. The first step in treating device-related perforation is to make sure there is adequate wire across the lesion and to promptly perform a low-pressure balloon inflation across the ruptured vessel. The balloon size should be 1 to 1 with the vessel lumen at the site of rupture and typically long enough to straddle the perforated segment. The balloon is kept inflated for 3–5 min at 2–4 atmospheres. If possible, angiography may be performed to confirm that the balloon is completely sealing the perforation. If the complication did not resolve, repeat balloon inflation may be performed especially if the perforation is getting resolved. Many operators will elect to reverse the anticoagulation however; this may not be possible with some anticoagulants such as bivalirudin or in some cases that require prolonged balloon inflation which may cause distal vessel thrombosis thus converting one bad complication into two. If balloon tamponade is not sufficient to seal a perforation, then a covered stent may be needed. Similar to other types of stents, there are two types of covered stents self-expanding (such as the Viabahn or WallFlex covered stent) and balloon expandable (such as the iCAST or LIFESTREAM covered stent). In general, self-expanding covered stents are used in the infrainguinal and external iliac vessels, and balloon-expandable stents are used

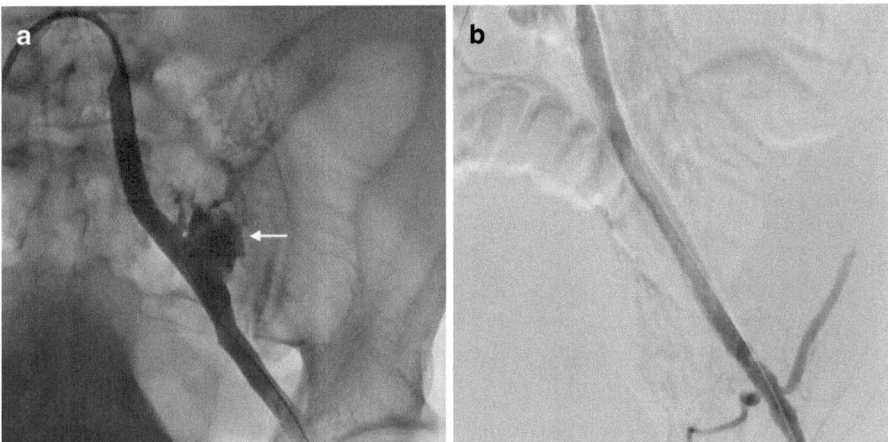

Fig. 7.11 Rupture of the iliac artery after postdilating the stent that was implanted to revascularize a totally occluded common iliac and external iliac artery. The contrast was free flowing into the retroperitoneal space (arrow) (**a**), and the patient developed hypotension within seconds. A balloon was used to tamponade the perforation, and a balloon-expandable covered stent was used to successfully seal the perforation (**b**)

in the common iliacs and distal aorta. The coronary balloon-expandable GRAFTMASTER or JOMED JOSTENT may be used in the infrapopliteal vessels. When using covered stents, it is important to decide on the appropriate stent diameter and length to avoid overstretching the vessel further and avoid occluding important side branches such as the internal iliac artery. At the same time, it is critical to completely cover the perforation to seal it off completely. In some cases, the patient may require surgical intervention to obtain hemostasis, but this is rare in the current era.

7.5.2 Dissections

Arterial dissections during peripheral interventions can be divided into three main categories. The first is the access site-related dissections. These, in general, are retrograde dissections that may be tacked up by the antegrade blood flow in that vessel (Fig. 7.12). If there is no pressure gradient across the dissection and it is small in size, one may elect to be conservative and follow up the dissection by noninvasive testing. One important aspect during the evaluation of such dissections is the fact that the pressure gradient as well as the angiographic appearance may be mild if there is a wire across the vessel that is holding the dissection flap. It may be important to evaluate the dissection after the wire is removed to make sure it does not transform into a hemodynamically significant dissection. In cases

Fig. 7.12 External iliac artery retrograde dissection (*arrow*), which is caused either due to the tip of the sheath that is against the wall of the artery (*star*) or due to the wire going subintimal after exiting the sheath

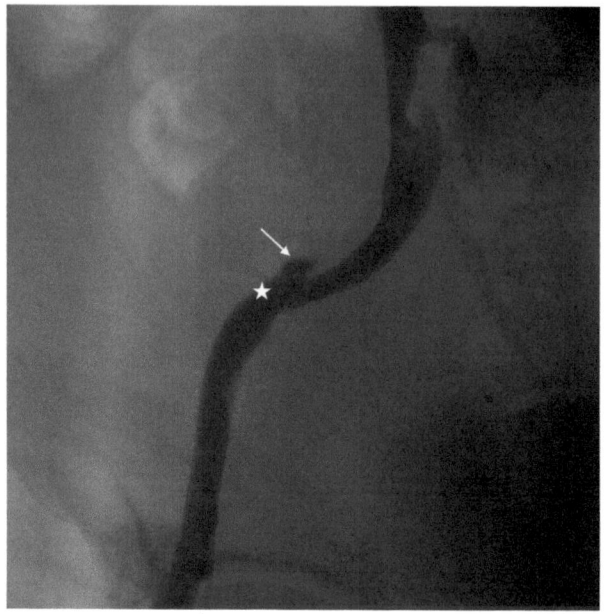

where the dissection is compromising blood flow to the distal extremity, stenting with a self-expanding stent may be necessary. If the dissection is severe and involves the CFA, surgery is the treatment of choice in order to prevent stenting across that vessel.

The second type of dissection occurs at the site of angioplasty of the vessel being treated. This is very common and in general does not require additional treatment unless the dissection is flow limiting. In such cases, additional treatment with stent placement is sufficient. Other treatment modalities such as surgery or prolonged balloon inflations may be needed for dissections in CFAs and popliteal artery if stenting is not desired or not an option. The third types of dissections are antegrade dissections, which may propagate due to blood flow across them. These will necessitate treatment in the majority of cases. Treatment is mainly with stenting, and this can be easily achieved if a wire is already across the lesion. However, if there is no wire across the lesion or the wire is lost during the intervention, it may be difficult to rewire across the dissected segment especially if there is a spiral dissection or the flow is completely occluded. In such cases, alternative access may be required to approach the dissection from a retrograde fashion or subintimal dissection, and reentry techniques may be used to reenter the true lumen and stent across the dissected segment. Surgery to fix such a complication is rarely needed with the current equipment and techniques that are being used.

7.5.3 Distal Embolization

Distal embolization (DE) of plaque or thrombus material during peripheral interventions may cause limb ischemia and sometimes worsen the clinical presentation especially in patients with critical limb ischemia. DE may occur during guidewire crossing, atherectomy, balloon angioplasty, and stent deployment (Fig. 7.13). In a retrospective analysis of 2137 lesions treated in 1029 patients with multiple modalities, the embolization rate was 1.6% [35]. In the same analysis, the embolization rate was significantly higher in TASC II C and D compared to TASC A and B lesions as well as for in-stent restenosis and CTO lesions compared to stenotic lesions. In addition, the Jetstream Pathway and Diamondback 360 devices had a significantly higher distal embolization rate (22%) as compared to balloon angioplasty alone (0.9%), balloon and stent (0.7%), SilverHawk (1.9%), and laser atherectomy (3.6%) [35]. It is important to mention that patency was restored in 94% of the patients that had distal embolization during the same procedure. There was no difference in the clinical outcome between patients with DE and those without.

In general, a distal runoff angiography should be performed after percutaneous revascularization of any vascular bed to evaluate for evidence of DE. Angiographic predictors of DE include CTO; long, irregular, and calcified lesions; as well as thrombotic occlusions. Distal embolization is mainly divided into two different types, micro- and macro-embolization. The clinical manifestation of either kind depends on the burden of material embolized and the vascular bed affected by the embolization. While such embolization may be catastrophic in the coronary or cerebral circulation, most of the time, it is of no clinical significance in the lower extremities. A major difference between micro- and macro-embolization is that in patient with micro-embolization, the capillary beds will get obstructed and collateral flow will not help the overall outcome and clinical picture. On the other hand, collateral flow may preserve a limb in cases with macro-embolization.

Prevention of DE may be the best treatment strategy. Although there are no prospective randomized data to support its use, and there are no devices approved for infrainguinal use, embolic protection devices (EPDs) are being used by many operators for that purpose especially with thrombectomy devices. Data from a number of small heterogeneous series of patients where EPDs were used during lower extremity interventions suggest that DE is very common in such interventions especially with atherectomy device usage and that the majority of DE occur during the procedure for acute and subacute lesions [36]. Filter clotting may result in cessation of distal flow, limiting angiographic assessment of the runoff vessels. Furthermore, EPD does not protect proximal collateral vessels, and the device itself may cause arterial spasm, injury, or de novo thrombus formation [37, 38].

A number of treatment strategies are possible in case of DE. Strategies differ depending on the type of DE and the duration since onset. Aspiration embolectomy, thrombolysis (if no contraindications), balloon angioplasty and stenting, open

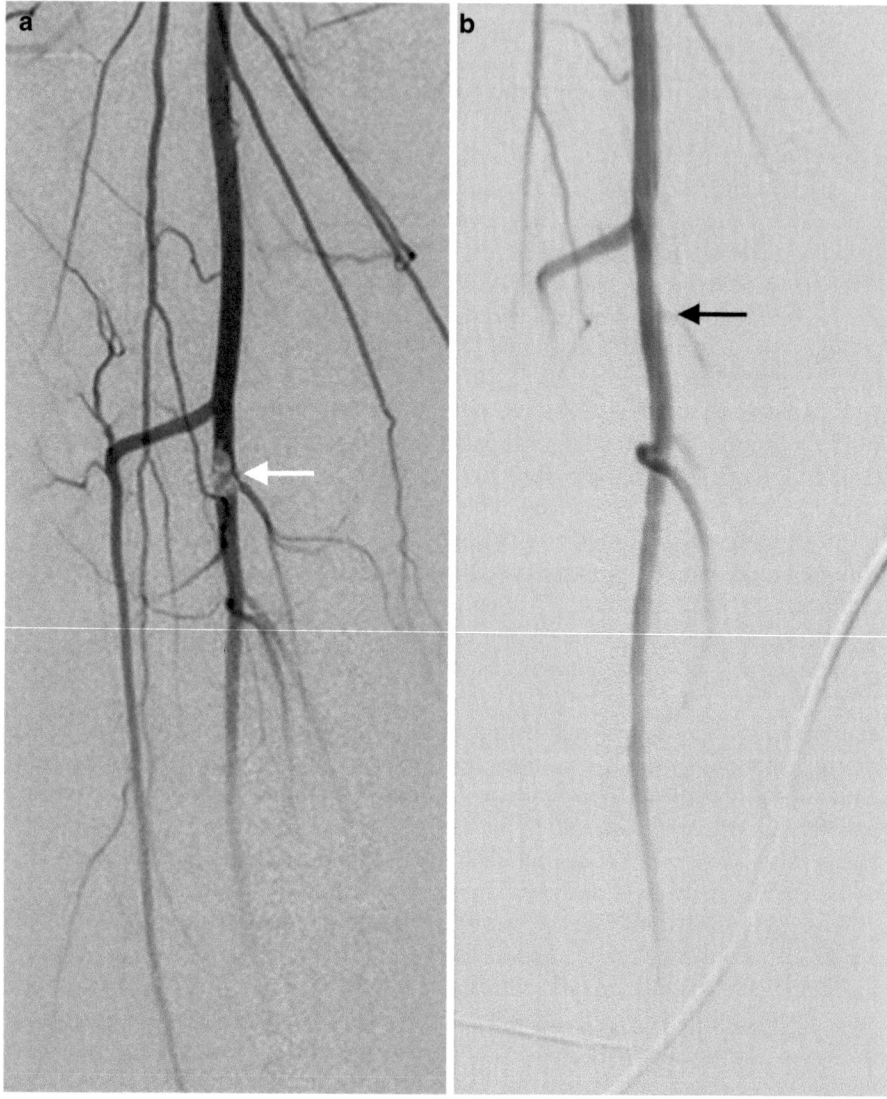

Fig. 7.13 After revascularization of the distal aorta, a runoff was performed, and distal emboliza-tion to the tibioperoneal trunk was noted (*white arrow*) with decrease perfusion of the distal arter-ies (**a**). Multiple attempts were made to aspirate the atheroma but were not successful so a stent was placed successfully across the embolized material (*black arrow*) (**b**)

surgical thrombectomy, or any combinations are all possible treatment options. The choice between endovascular treatments vs. open surgical options depends on the etiology and location of the occlusion as well as general contraindications to surgi-cal revascularization and/or the use of lytic agents.

7.5.4 Blue Toe Syndrome

Blue toe syndrome (Fig. 7.14) is caused by occlusion of small- and medium-caliber arteries (100–200 μm in diameter) by cholesterol and may be a complication of peripheral intervention. Cholesterol embolism is a challenge to diagnose and treat effectively. Livedo reticularis in the presence of good peripheral pulses is the most common skin manifestation of cholesterol embolism and is seen in 50–75% of skin lesions [39]. Other skin findings include necrosis and acrocyanosis or blue toe syndrome. The diagnosis is usually made clinically, and the provider should have a high index of suspicion especially in patients who had a recent instrumentation of the systemic circulation. This happens due to events or procedures that disrupt unstable atherosclerotic plaques, most frequently during invasive vascular procedures, and the administration of anticoagulants or thrombolytics. The most common sites for severe atherosclerotic disease are the abdominal aorta and the iliac and femoral arteries thus making interventions on the lower extremities an important iatrogenic cause blue toe syndrome.

Cholesterol crystals are showered into the bloodstream and migrate distally until they lodge in small arterioles. This causes an acute inflammatory response which in

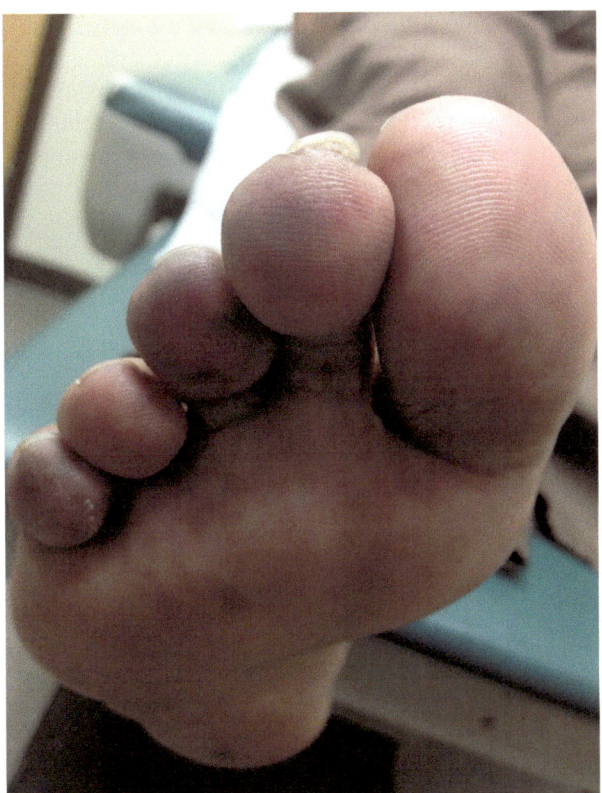

Fig. 7.14 Blue toe syndrome seen in a patient after iliac artery intervention

turn triggers a cascade of events leading to intravascular thrombus formation, endothelial proliferation, and, eventually, vessel fibrosis. Clinical manifestations may be immediate or a delay of several months. A study by Belenfant et al. of patients with cholesterol emboli found that the precipitating event occurred an average of 2 months prior to recognition of fulminant disease [40]. Cholesterol emboli may also cause a variety of other clinical manifestations including systemic, renal, gastrointestinal, and others which are beyond the scope of discussion of this book chapter. Patients with cholesterol emboli develop eosinophilia within few days, and the levels may remain elevated for up to a month. Treatment options are limited, and data is conflicting about some therapeutic approaches such as anticoagulation. In general, withholding all anticoagulation and thrombolysis if possible is helpful even though there are some reports of treating cholesterol emboli with anticoagulation. Do not attempt further endovascular procedures to decrease the risk of further cholesterol embolization. Long-term high-dose statins is important and modifying other risk factors.

7.6   Conclusion

Endovascular procedures have come a long way in terms of safety, efficacy, and procedural success rate. Like with any other invasive procedure, complications will occur, and some may cause significant morbidity and even mortality. While relatively rare, early diagnosis and treatment of complications during interventions of the lower extremity arterial beds remains critical to save limbs and lives. Perhaps the best treatment strategy is prevention by paying careful attention to procedural details as well as pre- and post-procedural care and planning.

References

1. Mohammad A, Banerjee A, Baig M, et al. TCT-352: angiographic features of atherosclerotic superficial femoral artery disease in diabetics and non-diabetics presenting with claudication. J Am Coll Cardiol. 2012;60(17_S):B100.
2. Scheinert D, Grummt L, Piorkowski M. A novel self-expanding interwoven nitinol stent for complex femoropopliteal lesions: 24-month results of the SUPERA SFA registry. J Endovasc Ther. 2011;18:745–52.
3. Abu-Fadel MS, Sparling JM, Zacharias SJ, et al. Fluoroscopy vs. traditional guided femoral arterial access and the use of closure devices: a randomized controlled trial. Catheter Cardiovasc Interv. 2009;74(4):533–9.
4. Ellis S, Bhatt D, Kapadia S, et al. Correlates and outcomes of retroperitoneal hemorrhage complicating percutaneous coronary intervention. Catheter Cardiovasc Interv. 2006;67:541–5.
5. Rupp S, Vogelzang R, Nemcek A, et al. Relationship of the inguinal ligament to pelvic radiographic landmarks: anatomic correlation and its role in femoral arteriography. J Vasc Interv Radiol. 1993;4:409–13.

6. Cilingiroglu M, Feldman T, Salinger M, et al. Fluoroscopically-guided micropuncture femoral artery access for large-caliber sheath insertion. J Invasive Cardiol. 2011;23(4):157–61.
7. Ben-Dor I, Maluenda G, Mahmoudi M, et al. A novel, minimally invasive access technique versus standard 18-gauge needle set for femoral access. Catheter Cardiovasc Interv. 2012;79:1180–5.
8. Seto AH, Abu-Fadel MS, Sparling JM, et al. Real-time ultrasound guidance facilitates femoral arterial access and reduces vascular complications: FAUST (Femoral Arterial Access With Ultrasound Trial). JACC Cardiovasc Interv. 2010;3:751–8.
9. Saha S, Gibson M, Magee T, et al. Early results of retrograde transpopliteal angioplasty of iliofemoral lesions. Cardiovasc Intervent Radiol. 2001;24:378–82.
10. Wiechmann B. Tibial intervention for critical limb ischemia. Semin Interv Radiol. 2009;26(4):315–23.
11. Pancholy S, Coppola J, Patel T, et al. Prevention of radial artery occlusion patent hemostasis evaluation trial (PROPHET study): a randomized comparison of traditional versus patency documented hemostasis after transradial catheterization. Catheter Cardiovasc Interv. 2008;72:335–40.
12. Sanmartin M, Cuevas D, Goicolea J, et al. Vascular complications associated with radial artery access for cardiac catheterization. Rev Esp Cardiol. 2004;57:581–4.
13. Tizon-Marcos H, Barbeau GR. Incidence of compartment syndrome of the arm in a large series of transradial approach for coronary procedures. J Interv Cardiol. 2008;21:380–4.
14. Hessel S, Adams D, Abrams H. Complications of angiography. Radiology. 1981;138:273–81.
15. Katzenschlager R, Ugurluoglu A, Ahmadi A, et al. Incidence of pseudoaneurysm after diagnostic and therapeutic angiography. Radiology. 1995;195:463–6.
16. Dzijan-Horn M, Langwieser N, Groha P. Safety and efficacy of a potential treatment algorithm by using manual compression repair and ultrasound-guided thrombin injection for the management of iatrogenic femoral artery pseudoaneurysm in a large patient cohort. Circ Cardiovasc Interv. 2014;7:207–15.
17. Shoulders-Odom B. Management of patients after percutaneous coronary interventions. Crit Care Nurse. 2008;28(5):26–41.
18. Nasser T, Mohler E, Wilensky R, et al. Peripheral vascular complications following coronary interventional procedures. Clin Cardiol. 1995;18(11):609–14.
19. Stone PA, Campbell JE. Complications related to femoral artery access for transcatheter procedures. Vasc Endovasc Surg. 2012;46(8):617–23.
20. Kim D, Orron D, Skillman J. Role of superficial femoral artery puncture in the development of pseudoaneurysm and arteriovenous fistula complicating percutaneous transfemoral cardiac catheterization. Catheter Cardiovasc Diagn. 1992;25(2):91.
21. Lamar R, Berg R, Rama K. Femoral arteriovenous fistula as a complication of percutaneous transluminal coronary angioplasty: a report of five cases. Am Surg. 1990;56(11):702.
22. Glaser R, McKellar D, Scher K. Arteriovenous fistulas after cardiac catheterization. Arch Surg. 1989;124(11):1313.
23. Fellmeth B, Roberts A, Bookstein J, et al. Postangiographic femoral artery injuries: nonsurgical repair with US-guided compression. Radiology. 1991;178(3):671.
24. Coppola J, Staniloae C. Radial access for peripheral vascular procedures. Endovasc Today. 2012;11(1):38–44.
25. Shammas N. Complications in peripheral vascular interventions: emerging role of direct thrombin inhibitors. J Vasc Interv Radiol. 2005;16:165–71.
26. Omran J, Firwana B, Duang V, et al. Hemorrhagic and ischemic outcomes of heparin vs. bivalirudin in carotid artery stenting: a meta-analysis of clinical trials. Catheter Cardiovasc Interv 2015;85(6):941–1107, E163–71.
27. Arora S, Panaich S, Patel N. Impact of hospital volume on outcomes of lower extremity endovascular interventions (insights from the nationwide inpatient sample [2006 to 2011]). Am J Cardiol. 2015;116(5):791–800.

28. Swee W, Wang J, Lee A. Managing perforations of the superficial femoral artery. Endovasc Today. 2014;13(10):59–68.
29. Lewis DR, Bullbulia RA, Murphy P, et al. Vascular surgical intervention for complications of cardiovascular radiology: 13 years' experience in a single centre. Ann R Coll Surg Engl. 1999;81:23–6.
30. Hayes P, Chokkalingam A, Jones R. Arterial perforation during infrainguinal lower limb angioplasty does not worsen outcome: results from 1409 patients. J Endovasc Ther. 2002;9:422–7.
31. McKinsey J, Zeller T, Rocha-Singh K, et al. Lower extremity revascularization using directional atherectomy: 12-month prospective results of the DEFINITIVE LE study. JACC Cardiovasc Interv. 2014;7:923–33.
32. Laird J, Zeller T, Gray B, et al. Limb salvage following laser-assisted angioplasty for critical limb ischemia: results of the LACI multicenter trial. J Endovasc Ther. 2006;13:1–11.
33. Zeller T, Krankenberg H, Steinkamp H, et al. One-year outcome of percutaneous rotational atherectomy with aspiration in infrainguinal peripheral arterial occlusive disease. J Endovasc Ther. 2009;16:653–62.
34. Lee MS, Yang T, Adams G. Pooled analysis of the CONFIRM registries: safety outcomes in diabetic patients treated with orbital atherectomy for peripheral artery disease. J Endovasc Ther. 2014;2:258–65.
35. Shrikhande G, Khan S, Hussain H, et al. Lesion types and device characteristics that predict distal embolization during percutaneous lower extremity interventions. J Vasc Surg. 2011;53:347–52.
36. Brancaccio G, Lombardi R, Stefanini T, et al. Comparison of embolic load in femoropopliteal interventions: percutaneous transluminal angioplasty versus stenting. Vasc Endovasc Surg. 2012;46(3):229–35.
37. Konig C, Pusich B, Tepe G, et al. Frequent embolization in peripheral angioplasty: detection with an embolism protection device (AngioGuard) and electron microscopy. Cardiovasc Intervent Radiol. 2003;26(4):334–9.
38. Karnabatidis D, Katsanos K, Kagadis G, et al. Distal embolism during percutaneous revascularization of infra-aortic arterial occlusive disease: an underestimated phenomenon. J Endovasc Ther. 2006;13(3):269–80.
39. Jucgla A, Moreso F, Muniesa C, et al. Cholesterol embolism: still an unrecognized entity with a high mortality rate. J Am Acad Dermatol. 2006;55(5):786–93.
40. Belenfant X, Meyrier A, Jacquot C. Supportive treatment improves survival in multivisceral cholesterol crystal embolism. Am J Kidney Dis. 1999;33(5):840–50.